Integrating Faith and Science through Natural Family Planning

Integrating Faith and Science through Natural Family Planning

Richard J. Fehring, D.N.Sc., R.N.
Theresa Notare, M.A.
Editors

Marquette University Press

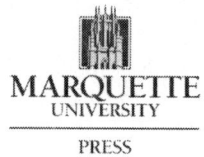

MARQUETTE
UNIVERSITY
PRESS

Library of Congress Cataloguing-in-Publication Data

Integrating faith and science through natural family planning / Richard J. Fehring, Theresa Notare, editors.—1st ed.
  p. ; cm.
Includes bibliographical references and index.
ISBN 0-87462-011-2 (pbk. : alk. paper)
1. Natural family planning. 2. Birth control—Religious aspects—Catholic Church. 3. Religion and science.
[DNLM: 1. Natural Family Planning Methods—Congresses. 2. Catholicism—Congresses. 3. Religion and Science--Congresses.] I. Fehring, Richard J., 1948- II. Notare, Theresa, 1957-
RG136.5.I53 2004
613.9'434—dc22

2004002834

© Marquette University Press 2004
All rights reserved.

Marquette University Press
Member, American Association of University Presses
Association of Jesuit University Presses

Cover photo of the trumeau sculpture of Adam and Eve with baby,
west façade, south portal of Amiens Cathedral
by Andew J. Tallon

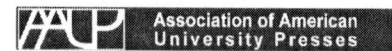

MARQUETTE UNIVERSITY PRESS
MILWAUKEE

The Association of Jesuit University Presses

Table of Contents

Foreword

Integrating Faith and Science through Natural Family Planning: Forward and Overview to the Proceedings.................................... 9
Richard J. Fehring, D.N.Sc., R.N. Professor, Marquette University
Theresa Notare, M.A. Assistant Director, Diocesan Developmen Program for Natural Family Planning, United States Conference of Catholic Bishops

Keynote Address

Integrating Faith & Science through NFP 15
Most Rev. Daniel Buechlein, O.S.B., D.D. Archbishop of Indianapolis

Theme: Spiritual Foundations of NFP

NFP and Marital Spirituality 29
John Grabowski, Ph.D. Catholic University of America
Respondent: Mark Johnson, Ph.D. Marquette University 46

A Feminist Perspective of NFP and Contraception
Theresa Wagner, J.D. Washington DC 49
Respondent: Cynthia Jones-Nosacek, M.D. Columbia–St.Mary's, Milwaukee, WI 62

The Future of Obstetrics and Gynecology: The Right to be Trained & Practice According to Conscience 71
Hanna Klaus, M.D. NFP Center of Washington D.C.
Respondent: James Linn, M.D. Columbia–St.Mary's, Milwaukee, WI 76

Theme: Scientific Foundations of NFP

Day-Specific Probabilities of Conception in the Menstrual Cycle
Joseph B. Stanford, M.D., M.S.P.H. University of Utah and David B. Dunson, Ph.D. National Institute of Environmental Health Sciences, Research Triangle, North Carolina 79

Perimenopause: Physiological Parameters
Nancy Reame, Ph.D., R.N. Professor, University of Michigan
Stages of Reproductive Aging Workshop (STRAW) 101
See Appendix 1 269
Respondent: Kathleen M. Raviele, M.D., F.A.C.O.G. Private Practice, Atlanta, GA 102

Efficacy of a new method of family planning:
the Standard Days Method
Marcos Arevalo, M.D., M.P.H., Victoria Jennings, Ph.D., and Irit Sinai, Ph.D., Georgetown University 107
See Appendix 2 275
Respondent: Joseph B. Stanford, M.D., M.S.P.H 108

Psychological Aspects of Achieving or Avoiding Pregnancy
Lawrence J. Severy, Ph.D. University of Florida–Gainesville and Janet Robinson, Family Health International, Research Triangle Park, North Carolina 111
Respondent: Richard J. Fehring, D.N.Sc., R.N. Marquette University 134

Correlates of Marital Satisfaction in a Sample of NFP Women
Andrew C. Pollard, State University of New York at Buffalo, and Mercedes Arzú-Wilson, Family of the Americas Foundation, Dunkiak, M.D. 139
Respondent: Julie Krause, B.S.N., R.N. Diocese of Madison, WI 166

Contents

Preliminary Comparison of Algorithm-Interpreted Fertility Monitor Readings with Established Natural Family Planning Methods
Jennine Regas, M.S. and Philip Regas, M.B.A. Zetek, Inc., Aurora, CO 169
Respondent: Barbara Savinetti–Rose, R.N., M.S.N. Philadelphia, PA 178

Undergirding Abstinence within a Sexuality Education Program
Hanna Klaus, M.D., Mary Nora Dennehy, and Jean Turnbull 183
Respondent: Alice B. Heinzen, M.A., Diocese of La Crosse, WI.... 201

A Life History Study of Sexually Abstinent, Adolescent, African American Females
Kristin Haglund R.N., Ph.D., Marquette University 203

Comparison of Ecological Breastfeeding with Lactation Amenorrhea Method (LAM)
Sheila Matgen Kippley, Couple to Couple League International, Cincinnati, OH 215

Abstract from Poster Presentation

Arguments Against Contraception–Do They Make Sense to the General Public? Importance of ethics, religion and "natural morality" in choice of family planning methods
Rafael Mikolajczyk, M.D., Otto-von-Guericke-University of Magdeburg, Magdeburg, Germany, and Joseph Stanford, M.D., University of Utah 227

Pre-conference Workshop on the Ovarian Monitor

Introduction to the Ovarian Monitor and Applications for Assessment Practice and Research
Leonard F. Blackwell, Ph.D., Massey University, Palmerston North, New Zealand 231

Eavesdropping on the Ovary. Hormonal Correlates of Fertility in the Human Menstrual Cycle
Leonard F. Blackwell, Ph.D., Massey University, Palmerston North, New Zealand 247

Appendix 1: *Stages of Reproductive Aging Workshop* (STRAW) 266

Appendix 2: *Efficacy of a new method of family planning: the Standard Days Method* 271

Index 277

Integrating Faith and Science through Natural Family Planning
Forward and Overview to the Proceedings

Richard J. Fehring, D.N.Sc., R.N.
Professor, Marquette University

Theresa Notare, M.A.
Assistant Director, Diocesan Development Program for Natural Family Planning, United States Conference of Catholic Bishops

The title of these proceedings is taken from a conference that was sponsored by Marquette University College of Nursing Institute for Natural Family Planning and the Diocesan Development Program for Natural Family Planning, Secretariat for Pro-Life Activities, United States Conference of Catholic Bishops. The conference was held at Marquette University in Milwaukee, Wisconsin on June 20-22, 2002 and included national and international scholars that represented health care, science, law and theology. The purpose of the conference was to explore the integration of faith and science through natural family planning (NFP). In keeping with the purpose, the format of the conference was divided into two days and two themes: day one on the theme, *Spiritual Foundations of NFP* and day two on the theme, *Scientific Foundations of NFP.* The conference started with a keynote presentation by Most Rev. Daniel M. Buechlein, O.S.B., Archbishop of Indianapolis. Archbishop Buechlein provided an overview of the connections between faith and science. His presentation included topics such as the value of chastity for the holistic health of the human person, the Church's understanding of family planning, and the interplay of NFP with science.

The Spiritual Foundations of NFP was explored on day one of the conference. John Grabowski, Ph.D., Associate Dean of Religious

Studies, Catholic University of America, provided the theological framework for how NFP can integrate and sanctify marital life. Using sources from the contemporary life of the Church, Dr. Grabowski argued that the "practice of NFP can foster a couple's capacity to live their marital consecration to holiness sharing in Christ's mission as priest, prophet, and king not only through periodic continence but also through making more authentic the bodily gifts of themselves in their sexual union." Mark Johnson, Ph.D., Assistant Professor, Department of Theology, Marquette University, responded to Dr. Grabowski's paper.

Theresa Wagner, Esq., provided a feminist perspective of NFP and contraception. Ms. Wagner, a lobbyist from Washington, D.C., provided conference participants with an overview of the type of legal battles that pro-life feminists have waged in government. The context was especially important in order to understand the kinds of values which are currently at stake in the United States. Ms. Wagner saw much hope in the practice of NFP, calling it more than "fertility awareness." "NFP," she said, "promotes appreciation of female fertility—ultimately—appreciation of the women. How we treat the women's cycle tells us something about our attitude toward women." Cindy Jones-Nosacek, M.D. gave a personal response to Ms. Wagner's presentation by providing her view of how she as a woman and NFP only physician is treated in a society that often views fertility and women not as gift but rather as objects.

The first full day of the conference ended with remarks on the topic, "The Future of Obstetrics and Gynecology: The Right to be Trained and Practice According to Conscience," by Hanna Klaus, M.D., Executive Director of the NFP Center of Washington, DC. Dr. Klaus had attended a Vatican sponsored program on the same topic. Her respondents included two other NFP only obstetricians and gynecologists, Julie Mickelson, M.D. and James Linn, M.D., both of Columbia-St. Mary's Hospital, Milwaukee, Wisconsin.

Day two of the conference focused on the scientific foundations of NFP. The day started with a paper presented by Joseph Stanford, M.D., Associate Professor in the Department of Family and Preventive Medicine at the University of Utah, and written with David Dunson, Ph.D., Research Fellow, National Institutes of Environmental Health

Sciences. Their paper on the day specific probabilities of fecundity is a summarization of current research in that area. Of particular interest was the latest research on the effects of aging in the decline of fertility among both women and men. Nancy Reame, Ph.D., R.N., Professor, University of Michigan, presented some of the physiological reasons for the decline of fertility among peri-menopausal women. Dr. Reame included information in her paper on a new consensus model and definition for the process of peri-menopause. The model represents an executive summary from the *Stages of Reproductive Aging Workshop*. Called the STRAW staging system, the executive summary is reproduced with permission in these proceedings. Kathleen Raviele, M.D., an NFP only obstetrician and gynecologist from Atlanta, provided a response from a clinician's view to Dr. Reame's presentation.

The afternoon of the second day began with a presentation by Larry Severy, Ph.D. Professor of Psychology, University of Florida at Gainesville. His paper analyzed the psychological acceptance of new methods of family planning and presented psychological data on the use of new technology that has been developed to help couples both achieve and avoid pregnancy. The measurement tool that he developed to determine psychological acceptance includes indicators (such as communication) that could be used as a standardized way to evaluate the use of different methods of NFP. One of his clearest insights was that "one method of NFP does not fit all people." A new method of NFP called the Standard Day Method and implemented through the use of a bead system, was presented by Marcos Arevalo, M.D., Georgetown University Institute for Reproductive Health. Dr. Arevalo's paper discussed the results of an effectiveness study of the new method. Dr. Joseph Stanford provided an insightful response.

The conference ended with a scientific paper session that was moderated by Mary Lee Barron, M.S.N., C.F.N.P., Assistant Professor, St. Louis University. The papers for this session were selected by a call for abstracts. Included among the papers were: The Teen Star Program and its effects on delaying premature intercourse, by Hanna Klaus, M.D., Alice Heinzen, M.A., Diocesan NFP Co-coordinator, La Crosse, Wisconsin, responded; marital satisfaction among women users of NFP using a sociological model for analyzing that data, by Andrew Pollard, Ph.D., Department of Sociology, The State University of New York at Buffalo, Julie Krause, R.N., Diocesan NFP Coordinator, Madison, Wisconsin, respondent; and an evaluation and comparison of the OvuQue fertility monitor with the methods of NFP, by Phillip Regas, M.S. and Jennine Regas, M.S, Zetek Inc, Aurora, Colorado, Barbara Rose, R.N, M.S.N., Philadelphia NFP Network, respondent.

Three additional papers were selected through the call for abstracts and were presented either during a lunch break or as a poster presentation. Kristin Haglund, Ph.D., R.N., Assistant Professor of Nursing, Marquette University, presented the results from her qualitative study on why African – American adolescent females remain and choose to be sexually abstinent. NFP pioneer and co-founder of the Couple to Couple League, Sheila Matgen Kippley, B.S. presented her experiences and perspectives on ecological breastfeeding in comparison to the Lactation Ammenorrhea Method (LAM). The final paper on the comparison of the reasons for rejecting contraception and using NFP between German and Polish women by Rafael Mikolajczyk, M.D, Otto-von-Guericke University, Magdeburg, Germany was presented as a poster.

Prior to this two day conference was a one day pre-conference presentation and workshop on the Ovarian Monitor by Len Blackwell, Ph.D., Associate Professor, Department of Chemistry, Massey University, New Zealand. Dr. Blackwell gave a brief overview of the balanced physiological process of human female reproductive hormones. He discussed the history and development of the Ovarian Monitor and described how the monitor could be used for assessment of the menstrual cycle as well as its application in an NFP practice. Finally, he discussed the monitor's potential use for research. Dr. Blackwell also described the computer data system that is being developed with the monitor and some of the hormonal profiles for various reproductive categories that are emerging from his work and other colleagues that are working with the Ovarian Monitor in conjunction with its inventor Dr. James Brown from Australia.

We believe that these proceedings will benefit the NFP community. We hope they will stimulate discussion, advance practice, research, and scholarship in NFP. Most of all, we hope the work presented here will act as a support to those who provide and promote NFP. The methods of Natural Family Planning are viable and moral forms of family planning. Indeed, they promote a *healthy way of life*. Finally, we hope that these proceedings demonstrate how faith and science can work together.

Acknowledgments

These proceedings would not be possible without the tireless help from Mary Schneider, B.S.N., R.N., Assistant to the Director of the Marquette University Institute for NFP. Ms. Schneider helped to obtain the completed manuscripts from the presenters, coordinated efforts between the publisher, writers and editors and obtained permissions from publishers to copy tables and reprint articles. We also wish to thank Janet Kistler, Special Assistant to the Diocesan Development Program for NFP, USCCB and Vivian Potemkin for assisting in reading and editing the manuscripts. Finally, we wish to thank Andrew Tallon, Ph.D., Director of Marquette University Press, and Maureen Kondrick, Manager of Marquette University Press, for their patience and assistance in producing these proceedings.

Richard J. Fehring, D.N.Sc., R.N.
Professor and Director, Institute for Natural Family Planning,
College of Nursing,
Marquette University

Theresa Notare, M.A.
Assistant Director, Diocesan Development Program for Natural Family Planning, Secretariat for Pro-Life Activities,
United States Conference of Catholic Bishops

Integrating Faith and Science through Natural Family Planning

Most Rev. Daniel M. Buechlein, O.S.B.
Archbishop of Indianapolis

1. The Reason We Are Here

The title for this conference would sound surprising to the ordinary person in the street. For historical reasons, some would be uncomfortable with the very idea of trying to integrate faith and science. Indeed, some would certainly be uncomfortable with the notion of Natural Family Planning, and they would be extremely uncomfortable at the mere suggestion that Natural Family Planning could be a point of integrating faith and science. Perhaps we should say from the outset that this discomfort is symptomatic of the present culture. The very expression of our theme is countercultural. Yet, we are here to explore precisely this theme of "integrating faith and science through Natural Family Planning."

Presumably it is my task to present the overview of the Catholic Church on the topic. I will do so in the following manner: In introductory fashion, I will sketch the current societal and ecclesial milieu in which our theme is viewed with discomfort, if indeed it is not simply ignored. Then briefly I will set forth the Church's vision of the relationship of faith and science. Second, I will present the Church's position on Natural Family Planning in the context of our Faith. Third, I will present our ecclesial view of the intersecting relationship of Natural Family Planning and science. The primary sources for much of what I say will be the document of the Second Vatican Council on *The Church in the Modern World* (*Gaudium et spes*) and the *Catechism of the Catholic Church.*

2. The Contemporary View of Faith and Science

In a largely secular view of human life and culture, faith is considered something very individual and largely self-serving. Religious faith is viewed as passé by some, or perhaps it is viewed as something needed by the less sophisticated or less educated members of our society. Some embrace the Marxist view that religion is "the opiate" of the people. At best, faith belongs in a different world and as such is best left unrelated to science. In this view, religion is considered a potential obstacle to human progress.

From another perspective, people rightly view science as the road and means to progress for the human family. Many members of contemporary society would subscribe to the principle that whatever scientific progress is possible should be pursued. If scientific technology fosters convenience and pleasure and financial profit, by that very fact some would maintain that it is a good to be pursued. For some, morality or ethical consideration of scientific advances is of secondary concern at best. For some, scientific progress is the only road to progress and the well-being of human society. As a religious leader and as a pastor, I submit that we are addressing a complex topic that is considered controversial and unpopular because many people "do not know what they do not know." And in our current culture, it is difficult to get a hearing on this theme in order to bring more light to the value both of the relationship of faith and science and of Natural Family Planning itself. And so, in the name of many other leaders of faith, I bring an expression of gratitude to the planners and sponsors of this conference.

I think we would agree that many are not interested in relating science and ecclesial faith because the concept conjures up memories such as the debacle concerning the Galileo controversy in the early Renaissance. The topic is further complicated in some circles by a misunderstanding of the Catholic Church's doctrine on infallibility.

In our current culture, artificial contraception as a means of family planning is simply a given for most married and unmarried people. Our Catholic population seems to mirror the wider culture. The institution of marriage has been losing ground to cohabitation instead of, or prior to, marriage. This phenomenon, and the movement in our culture to accept same-sex unions as marriages, are telling indicators of a diminishment of the traditional value of marriage and family life. Natural Family Planning in this context is viewed as virtually irrelevant and unwelcome.

It is also simply a fact that many people, Catholic priests and lay people alike, do not know that Natural Family Planning is the umbrella term for several natural, modern and scientific methods of family planning.

3. The Church's View of the Relationship between Faith and Science

Gaudium et spes (*Joy and Hope*) is the title of the Second Vatican Council document on *The Church in the Modern World*. In that document, the Catholic Church asserts that science can lay open new roads to truth and "elevate the human family to a more sublime understanding of truth, goodness and beauty, and to the formation of judgments which embody universal values" (*Gaudium et spes*, 57). The Church values the role of science for the betterment of the world (see *Gaudium et spes*, 5). In the view of the Church, "earthly matters and the concerns of faith derive from the same God" (*Gaudium et spes*, 36). Faith can provide science with the context in which to locate its discoveries, suggesting what is best for the human family and all of creation (see Notare 1994).

The *Catechism of the Catholic Church* addresses the relationship of faith and science by positing the common source of faith and science in these words:

> Though faith is above reason, there can never be any real discrepancy between faith and reason. Since the same God who reveals mysteries and infuses faith has bestowed the light of reason on the human mind, God cannot deny himself, nor can truth ever contradict truth. (*Dei Filius*, 4, DS 3017)
>
> Consequently, methodical research in all branches of knowledge, provided it is carried out in a truly scientific manner and does not override moral laws, can never conflict with the faith because the things of the world and things of faith derive from the same God. The humble and persevering investigator of the secrets of nature is being led, as it were, by the hand of God in spite of himself, for it

is God, the conserver of all things, who made them what they are. (*Gaudium et spes* 36, n. 1; quoted in the *Catechism*, 159)

Pertinent to our theme in this symposium, surely we can agree that faith and science intersect in their common concern for and common responsibility for the good of the human person as an individual, for the communal good of the human family, and for the significance and the good of human sexuality for both the individual and the human family.

4. Faith and the Catholic Church's Concern for Natural Family Planning

In an article on this topic that was published by our bishops' Secretariat for Pro-Life Activities in 1994, Theresa Notare wrote:

> It is no secret that some people question the Church's admonition against sexual intercourse outside of marriage, while others reject the teaching outright. In some circles it is acceptable—even politically correct—to mock the Church's beliefs. Yet the scientific study of human sexual behavior confirms the validity and the wisdom of Church teaching, and at the same time challenges us to respond to an emerging crisis. (Notare 1994, 2)

A. The Context: the Catholic Church's Vision of the Sacredness of Marriage and Family

Natural Family Planning, as the title implies, must be understood and evaluated in the context of the Church's vision of marriage and family in society. Realizing that our Church teaching about the sacrament of matrimony is voluminous, I will limit my words to those found in the Catechism of the Catholic Church, which treats of marriage extensively. The lead statement reads:

> The matrimonial covenant, by which a man and a woman establish between themselves a partnership of the whole of life, is by its nature ordered toward the good of the spouses and the procreation and education of offspring; this covenant between baptized persons has been raised by Christ the Lord to the dignity of a sacrament.

(*Code of Canon Law*, can.1055, n. 1; see *Gaudium et spes*, 48, n. 1; quoted in the *Catechism*, 1601)

The *Catechism* reminds us that marriage is not purely a human institution despite the variations it may have undergone through the centuries in many cultures. Some sense of the greatness of the conjugal union exists in all cultures. Quoting *Gaudium et spes*, the *Catechism* states: "The well-being of the individual person and of both human and Christian society is closely bound up with the healthy state of conjugal and family life' (n.1)" (*Catechism*, 1603).

The Church's vision of marriage includes concern for both the individual spouses and the family, for human society and Christian society. Marriage is not a private and individualistic state of life. Hence marriage is publicly witnessed, and it is blessed by a minister of the Church.

Spouses are consecrated and strengthened for their duties and the dignity of their state in the sacrament of matrimony. They are strengthened by God's grace. For coping with the challenges that test the sacred bond of marriage does not come naturally. Understanding the maturity required to live in the marital state with integrity and fidelity requires education and spiritual practices.

The *Catechism* speaks of the importance of the example of parents and families in preparing young people for marriage.

The role of pastors and of the Christian community as the 'family of God' is indispensable in the transmission of the human and Christian values of marriage and family and much more so in our era when many young people experience broken homes which no longer sufficiently assure this initiation:

It is imperative to give suitable and timely instruction to young people, above all in the heart of their own families, about the dignity of married love, its role and its exercise, so that, having learned the value of chastity, they will be able at a suitable age to engage in honorable courtship and enter upon a marriage of their own. (*Gaudium et spes*, 49, n. 3; quoted in the *Catechism*, 1632)

B. The Gift of Children

Implicit in the Catholic Church's regard for the married state and for family life is the understanding that children are the fruit of conjugal love, hence are viewed as a gift co-created by spouses and God. Children are viewed neither as a burden, nor as property to which spouses have the right of ownership. Gifts are freely given. On the other hand, "the refusal of fertility turns married life away from its 'supreme gift,' the child." (*Catechism*, 1664 quoting *Gaudium et spes* 50, n. 1).

C. The Church's Understanding of Human Sexuality

The Catholic Church understands responsibility for family and Natural Family Planning in relationship to her understanding of human sexuality. Theresa Notare succinctly describes the Church's vision of human sexuality as "scripturally based, sacramentally real, morally honest, and spiritually rich. In other words the Church promotes a holistic view of the human person—body, mind, and soul" (Notare 1994, 3).

"God is love and in himself he lives a mystery of personal loving communion. Creating the human race in his own image ... God inscribed in the humanity of man and woman the vocation, and thus the capacity and responsibility, of love and communion" (*Familiaris consortio*, 11). The capacity to love (and to procreate) is affected by the sexuality of the human person as it affects the unity of body and soul. The *Catechism* reminds us that sexuality especially concerns affectivity, the capacity to love and to procreate, and in a more general way the aptitude for forming bonds of communion with others (see *Catechism*, 2332). God gives man and woman an equal personal dignity as "both were created in the image and likeness of the personal God" (see *Catechism*, 2334).

The Catholic Church understands human sexuality as designed by God. This belief can be seen in the teaching of the *Catechism of the Catholic Church*. I quote extensively here because of the clarity of the text:

> Sexuality is ordered to the conjugal love of man and woman. In marriage the physical intimacy of the spouses becomes a sign and pledge of spiritual communion. Marriage bonds between baptized persons are sanctified by the sacrament. (*Catechism*, 2360)

Addressing our theme directly the *Catechism* states:

> The acts in marriage by which the intimate and chaste union of the spouses takes place are noble and honorable; the truly human performance of these acts fosters the self-giving they signify and enriches the spouses in joy and gratitude. (*Gaudium et spes*, 49, n. 2) Sexuality is a source of joy and pleasure. (*Catechism*, 2362)

The spouses' union achieves the twofold end of marriage: the good of the spouses themselves and the transmission of life. These two meanings or values of marriage cannot be separated without altering the couple's spiritual life and compromising the goods of marriage and the future of the family. "The conjugal love of man and woman thus stands under the twofold obligation of fidelity and fecundity (*Catechism*, 2363).

The Church has a profound respect for human sexuality and its essential connection with the bond of creative love of spouses in marriage. Separation from the creative love of married partners trivializes human sexuality, rendering it selfish and manipulative. The Church's vision of human sexuality promotes authentic freedom, the opportunity to grow in holiness and thus to experience profound peace.

D. The Value of Chastity for the Holistic Health of the Human Person

Charity is the form of all the virtues, and it is a measure of holistic maturity. Chastity is a virtue that safeguards and enhances generous and disinterested love. Chastity is the way to internal freedom because it is the means to maintain the integrity of the powers of life and love with which the human person is created. This integrity ensures the unity of the person. The *Catechism of the Catholic Church* states that chastity includes an apprenticeship in self-mastery which is a training in human freedom. The alternative is clear. The human person either governs his or her passions and finds peace, or is dominated by them and becomes unhappy. Self-mastery is a long and exacting work. One can never consider it acquired once and for all. It presupposes renewed effort in all stages of life (see *Catechism*, 2339, 2342).

Indeed, the practice of chastity requires the practice of ascetism in any state of life.

Chastity is an important tool for fostering generous conjugal love. It remains an eminently personal task in fostering the communion of spouses in genuine love. Spouses share the responsibility to look after the good of each other by remaining faithful to each other, and they share the responsibility for an openness to the transmission of life. Chastity is an essential aid to wife and husband.

E. The Church's Understanding of Family Planning

What about family planning? The *Catechism* asserts that

> Periodic continence, that is, the methods of birth regulation based on self-observation and the use of infertile periods, is in conformity with the objective criteria of morality (see *Humanae vitae*, 16). These methods respect the bodies of the spouses, encourage tenderness between them, and favor the education of an authentic freedom. In contrast, "every action which, whether in anticipation of the conjugal act, or in its accomplishment, or in the development of its natural consequences, proposes, whether as an end or as a means, to render procreation impossible" is intrinsically evil. (*Catechism*, 2370 quoting *Humanae vitae*,14)

Why, in the eyes of the Catholic Church, are artificial methods of family planning not morally and spiritually acceptable? The *Catechism* cites a clear statement of Pope John Paul II in his apostolic letter *Familiaris consortio*:

> Thus the innate language that expresses the total reciprocal self-giving of husband and wife is overlaid through contraception, by an objectively contradictory language, namely, that of not giving oneself totally to the other. This leads not only to a positive refusal to be open to life but also to a falsification of the inner truth of conjugal love, which is called upon to give itself in personal totality .... the difference, both anthropological and moral, between contraception and recourse to the rhythm of the cycle ... involves in the final analysis two irreconcilable concepts of the human person and of human sexuality. (*Familiaris consortio*, 32 quoted by the *Catechism*, 2370)

F. An Ecclesial View of the Stewardship of Creation

The creation account in Genesis tells us that, as God viewed his creation, he said it was good. In creating man and woman, God said "be fruitful and multiply." It is also clear from the Scriptures that man and woman are also called to be stewards of all creation. Concern for regulating births can be an important aspect of this stewardship. The Catholic Church understands this stewardship as mutual responsibility between spouses, responsibility to children as well as responsibility to society.

> The state has a responsibility for its citizens' well-being. In this capacity it is legitimate for it to intervene to orient the demography of the population. This can be done by means of objective and respectful information, but certainly not by authoritarian, coercive measures. The state may not legitimately usurp the initiative of spouses, who have the primary responsibility for the procreation and education of their children (see *Humanae vitae*, 23; *Populorum progressio*, 37). In this area, it is not authorized to employ means contrary to the moral law. (*Catechism*, 2372)

In her article, *Human Sexuality: Where Faith and Science Meet*, Theresa Notare writes that stewardship does not mean control at all costs.

> Responsibility and respect for creation are part of the reason why the Church cannot condone the use of artificial means to regulate births. The Church teaches that sexual intercourse is oriented to the future of our world. Fertility is a collective gift over which we have dominion but not absolute control. We need to understand and appreciate that God nourishes and renews the earth through his creative spirit. In this vision, fertility is not a problem for couples and the wider human family, but a gift and a mystery to be cherished, protected and respected. (Notare 1994, 3)

5. Natural Family Planning and Science

What do science and Natural Family Planning have in common? In a word, they intersect in mutual concern for the welfare of the human person. They are both concerned for the good of the individual human person and for the communal good of the human family as well.

From this viewpoint, science is concerned with human sexuality for a variety of reasons. There is cause to have grave concern because of the transmission of sexually related diseases in epidemic proportions. Science is concerned with issues related to the fertility of spouses. To some degree, science enters into the discussion about the demographic distribution of world population. As I indicated in my earlier remarks, the Church shares these concerns.

The Catholic Church's concern for the human person and the human family is holistic—that is, the Church holds the needs of body, mind and soul together. Both for the individual person and for society as a whole, the physical, psychological, moral and spiritual welfare are of a piece. The welfare of the human person and of human society is not served if the whole human person is not served. We believe that respect for the integrity of the ends of marriage is important for the welfare of the institution of marriage in society as well as for individual spouses. We believe that the psychological health of the individual person is deeply affected by whether the ends of marriage are respected in their totality. So is the welfare of the family in society.

The Catholic Church's concern for physical health in society is demonstrated by the enormous investment we have in health care both in sponsorship and services. I have already spoken of our respectful participation in a global concern for the stewardship of creation.

I do not think it is necessary to catalogue all the specific ways in which people of faith and scientists share a common concern for humanity for this audience. In general, we can say that we share a largely common purpose. Where science and faith differ is most often in the employment of means to the ends or purposes we hold in common.

Science enables society to make deeper connections between faith and our lives. Modern science has enabled Natural Family Planning methods to become more sophisticated and effective. The Sympto-Thermal Method, the Ovulation Method and the Basal Body Temperature Method are all scientifically based and make use of the observable signs of a woman's cycle of fertility.

A communications lag leaves too many people, including pastoral leaders, still skeptical about Natural Family Planning because of the Calendar Method of determining fertility, a method seldom used these days in the United States. This view of Natural Family Planning is scientifically inaccurate.

How effective is Natural Family Planning in our day? The World Health Organization and the U.S. Department of Health and Human Services both confirm a method effectiveness rate of 97-98 percent and an estimated user effectiveness of 85-95 percent.

Theresa Notare writes: "Research has helped the NFP community understand that in order for couples to achieve the 97-98 percent effectiveness rate, they must be taught by certified NFP instructors, be motivated to use the method, and be clear about their family intention" (Notare 1994, 4).

All of the literature I have perused on the topic of Natural Family Planning indicates that the most important factor for effectiveness is the intention of the couple using the method. Notare and others note that when couples are spacing births, they are more likely to disregard method rules and achieve the lower rates. In contrast, when couples have reached their family size they usually follow method rules more closely and achieve the higher rate.

Scientific data support the effectiveness of the natural method if the rules are followed and, as noted, intentionality makes all the difference. At the same time, there is in the world of science a pessimistic outlook about the ability of spouses to practice abstinence. It is precisely because some couples find abstinence during the monthly fertility period difficult that some in the medical profession do not encourage the methods of Natural Family Planning.

On the other hand, from the perspective of faith, the role of abstinence during the fertility cycle can be a positive factor. In fact from the perspective of faith, marital chastity is necessary in order to sustain a happy and fulfilling marriage.

Communication, mutual respect, responsible parenthood, enduring passion and mutual growth in faith are core components in married life. Natural Family Planning promotes a heightened awareness among couples that they must share their decision-making, and they must be concerned for their mutual responsibility for their behavior.

Communication in marriage is critical. Only through open communication do spouses grow in trust and respect for each other. Arriving at a mutual understanding of the precise intent of family planning promotes the health of marriage because it requires communication. Incidentally, NFP practitioners address this need for couples intending to use a Natural Family Planning method (see Sample 2001, 3-4).

The Church is aware of the challenge couples face in maintaining periodic abstinence when pursuing the natural method of family planning. Yet, looking at the totality of the human person and the totality of the challenge of communication and personal regard in marriage, the Church sees the abstinence and chastity required as a means to enhance conjugal love. Artificial contraception on the other hand permits, indeed tends to facilitate, a lack of open communication about discomforting fears or unarticulated values spouses may have. Artificial contraception not only allows relationships to be superficial, but also makes it easy to be manipulative, selfish and insensitive. It is not likely to foster intimacy that extends beyond the sexual arena.

From the perspective of faith, marital chastity and the value of periodic abstinence during the fertile time is likely to help spouses experience a mutual growth in faith as they use the natural method of family planning.

6. In Conclusion: Because There Is God

God is the creator of all that is good. It is the privilege of wife and husband to participate in God's creative act. It is not wholesome for humans to inadvertently or knowingly forget that in the end all is gift from God. Nor is it wholesome for spouses or the human family in general to forget about God and the Kingdom of God.

A year or so ago, for my birthday, one of my masters of ceremonies for confirmation gave me the first volume of Chicken Soup for the Soul. He said it might help my homilies.

I found a story about a little girl named Sachi and her new baby brother. After baby brother and mother came home from the hospital, Sachi kept asking her parents if she could spend some time alone with her new brother. Her parents worried that, as sometimes happens, Sachi might be a little jealous of the attention he was getting and, if left alone, might push him or something. Sachi kept asking. And her parents noticed that she was really very kind and gentle with her brother, so they said "ok." Sachi went to her brother's room and closed the door. Fortunately the door re-opened just a crack and her curious parents could not resist watching. Sachi went up to the crib, put her face close to her brother and said in a quiet voice: "Baby, what does God feel like? I am beginning to forget."

"What does God feel like? I'm beginning to forget." We do forget about God more easily than we would like, do we not? Perhaps when all is said and done our most important challenge is to remember that God is our creator and—ultimately—the giver of all that we have and are.

Bibliography

Canfield, Jack and Mark V. Hansen. 1993. *Chicken Soup for the Soul.* Vol.1. Health Communications, Inc.

Catechism of the Catholic Church. 1997. 2nd ed. Latin text by Libreria Editrice Vaticana, Citta del Vaticano, 1994 and 1997. English translation 1994 and 1997, Washington, D.C.: United States Catholic Conference.

Code of Canon Law (Codex Iuris Canonici). 1983. Translated under the auspices of the Canon Law Society of America. Washington, D.C.: Canon Law Society of America.

John Paul II. 1981. *Familiaris consortio (On the Role of the Christian Family in the Modern World).* Apostolic Exhortation.

Notare, Theresa. 1994. "Human Sexuality: Where Faith and Science Meet." *Respect Life Program.* Washington, D.C.: National Conference of Catholic Bishops, Secretariat for Pro-Life Activities.

Paul VI. 1968. *Humanae vitae (On the Regulation of Birth).* Encyclical.

———. 1967. *Populorum progressio (On the Development of Peoples).* Encyclical

Sample, Shelly. 2001. "Family Planning and Marital Chastity." *Ethics and Medics* 26: 3–4.

Vatican Council I. 1870. *Dei Filius (Dogmatic Constitution on the Catholic Faith).*

Vatican Council II. 1965. *Gaudium et spes (Pastoral Constitution on the Church in the Modern World).*

Natural Family Planning and Marital Spirituality

John S. Grabowski, Ph.D.
The Catholic University of America

Many commentators have pointed to the need for a distinctive "spirituality of marriage" in recent years (Parella 1982, 127-41; Örsy 1997, 38-54). Indeed, the Church itself in its recent teaching has emphasized the need for "a spirituality of motherhood and fatherhood" (John Paul II 1999, no. 46, p. 81). In many respects this observation seems to build upon the affirmation of the Second Vatican Council's *Lumen gentium* (nos. 39-42) that all in the Church are called to holiness and the perfection of charity (Abbott 1966, 65-72). If men and women who are married and the parents of children are called to holiness, then surely there must be some form of Christian life or some distinctive practices that can help them achieve it.

Unfortunately, models of marital spirituality are neither plentiful nor self-evident within the Church. The reasons for this are many and are largely embedded in the history of the Church's theological tradition. Early Christian pastors and theologians valued celibacy highly, based on the examples of Jesus and John the Baptist and the teaching of Paul (see 1 Cor. 7; Olsen 2001, 101-106). With the rise of monasticism in the fourth and fifth centuries, advocates of the ascetic life often placed marriage on the defensive. It seemed to many that marriage was antithetical to the real pursuit of holiness. The married might try to keep the Ten Commandments as best they could or if they did break them at least strive not to do so often, but many saw little hope for them to achieve genuine holiness (Mahoney 1987, 29). If any kind of spiritual life was offered to the married laity it often took the form of a watered down monasticism, so that the married might haltingly imitate their more committed and spiritual brethren. In either case, the clear impression often given was of a two-tiered spirituality: some were called to perfection, others to a less than immoral existence.

For many Christian monks and theologians the heart of the problem was the bodily nature of marriage and particularly the presence of sex within the marriage relationship. The pleasures of the flesh were too disruptive of human rationality—let alone of prayerful contemplation—to allow for progress in Christian virtue within marriage (e.g. the early Chrysostom's depiction of a married couple as two slaves chained together at the ankles each of whom impeded the other's spiritual progress by demanding sex in *De virginitate* 41.2). Even if such a relationship was faithful and procreative, continence was clearly viewed as better (Parella 1982, 132; dos Anjos 1995, 100). St. Augustine expressed the common viewpoint with straightforward economy: "continence from all intercourse is certainly better than marital intercourse itself which takes place for the begetting of children" (Augustine 1955, 17). This view lead some married couples to foreswear sexual relations altogether and to practice "spiritual marriage" (Elliott 1993). In our own day, the association of sex with dangerous forms of irrationality has undoubtedly been strengthened in the minds of some by the current scandal surrounding cases of clerical sexual misconduct—particularly the sexual abuse of minors.

Given the influence and pervasiveness of such views within the tradition and the dearth of models of marital spirituality in general, to suggest that something like natural family planning can actually shed light on or positively contribute to such a spirituality can seem to be more than a little quixotic. For even though for several decades the Church's magisterium has recommended natural methods of birth regulation as a morally licit alternative to contraception for those couples with serious reasons to avoid or postpone pregnancy, little theological attention has been devoted to the impact of these methods on a couple's shared spiritual life.

Yet there may be reason to think that this endeavor could be a fruitful one. For there are resources in its biblical and theological tradition and in the present teaching of the Church which point toward a spirituality of marriage capable of embracing the whole of married life. These same resources can serve to illuminate the significance of sexual union and abstinence as shaped by the use of NFP. It has been pointed out elsewhere that the periodic continence required by NFP facilitates the couple's growth in the virtue of chastity (Wojtyla 1993,

237-44). However, this paper will argue that the practice of NFP can foster a couple's capacity to live their marital consecration to holiness sharing in Christ's mission as priest, prophet, and king not only through the renunciation of periodic continence, but also through making more authentic the bodily gift of themselves in their sexual relationship. As such, it promotes an appreciation of the body and a balanced understanding of marital sexual expression as one integral dimension of the couple's call to communion.

To make this case this paper will first consider the foundation for a spirituality of marriage and sex within it in the baptismal sharing of the couple in the threefold mission of Christ. It will then relate in turn each of these dimensions of baptismal incorporation into Christ to the practice of NFP—priesthood, prophecy, and the kingship of mutual service. The conclusion will briefly consider the relevance of this analysis for larger questions of marital spirituality and its social significance.

Foundations for a Spirituality of Marriage

Echoing the teaching of the Second Vatican Council, the Apostolic Exhortation of Pope John Paul II *Christi fideles laici* emphasizes the baptismal sharing of the laity in the threefold mission of Christ. Citing *Lumen gentium* (no. 34), the document says of the priestly *mundus* of the laity,

> For their work, prayers, apostolic endeavors, their ordinary married and family life, their daily labor, their mental and physical relaxation, if carried out in the Spirit, and even the hardships of life if patiently born-all of these become spiritual sacrifices acceptable to God through Jesus Christ (1 Pt. 2:5). During the celebration of the Eucharist these sacrifices are most lovingly offered to the Father along with the Lord's body. Thus as worshipers whose every deed is holy, the lay faithful consecrate the world to God (John Paul II 1988, no. 41, p. 81).

It is noteworthy that all of the ordinary activities of marriage and family life, presumably including a couple's sexual relationship, are capable of being offered to God in the Church's eucharistic worship. As the source and summit of the Church's life (*Lumen gentium*, no.

11), the Eucharist is the chief source of its sanctification. As couples offer themselves and all of their day-to-day activities in the altar gifts of bread and wine, they like the gifts are transformed, becoming the Body of Christ acting in the world.

Joined to Christ, baptized men and women also share in his prophetic mission of proclaiming his Father's kingdom by their testimony to the gospel, by the witness of their lives, and by their resolute opposition to evil in all of its forms (see John Paul II 1988, no. 14, p. 31). Furthermore, "they are also called to allow the newness and power of the gospel to shine out everyday in their family and social life, as well as to express patiently and courageously in the contradictions of the present age their hope of future glory even 'through the framework of their secular life'" (John Paul II 1988, no. 14, p. 32). Hence the proclamation of Christian truth too should permeate the whole fabric of a couple's life—their work, recreation, community involvement, and interpersonal relationship. Certainly part of the couple's "resolute opposition to evil" should be the counter-cultural way they relate sexually in the midst of a culture, which trivializes sex to mere pleasure for the sake of personal fulfillment.

Finally, laymen and laywomen, in virtue of their baptism share in Christ's kingly mission and are called to be active agents of the spread of his Kingdom in history. They do this through opposition to the forces of evil in themselves and in the world, through concrete acts of justice and charity in which they touch the very person of Jesus present in the least of his brethren, and in ordering creation according to God's original plan for it (John Paul II 1988, no. 14, p. 32). The essence of this form of Christian kingship—as in the case of Jesus' own exercise of it—is its character of service. Such service, lived out in mutual deference of the spouses to one another is the very heart of marriage (Eph. 5:21-33; Grabowski 1997, 489-512). It is also central to the vocation of parenthood since fathers and mothers must continually place the needs of their children ahead of their own in decisions regarding the use of their time, their financial resources, and goals and priorities.

This sharing in the mission of Christ originates in and is sustained through the sacraments. It is founded in baptism, deepened by confirmation, and finds its "realization and dynamic sustenance in the

Holy Eucharist" (John Paul II 1988, no. 14, p. 33). Baptism changes Christians in their very being, conferring on them an ontological priesthood prior to the functional priesthood conferred by the sacrament of orders (Evdokimov 1995, 85-103). In the western understanding, this baptismal priesthood empowers men and women to confer the sacrament of marriage on one another (Örsy 1997, 45). Marriage in its own way deepens the couple's participation in Christ, consecrating them holiness in and through their life of fidelity and self-giving love (Rochetta 1997, 65-75). Spouses are thus given to one another as principal means to one another's holiness.

Numerous Church documents (e.g. *Lumen gentium*, no. 51, *Christifideles laici*, no. 15, *Ecclesia in America*, no. 44) refer to the distinctive mark of the lay vocation and hence of lay spirituality as "secularity." That is, this vocation is lived in the world and by this means the world is thus transformed and offered to its Creator. It is not in any sense a flight from the world as some have erroneously understood monasticism to comprise, but rather an embrace of a daily life lived in the world so that its "matter" might be consecrated by the word of the gospel. Marriage itself is a unique sign and participation in this reality, insofar as in it the natural love of a man and woman lived out in a myriad of ordinary gestures becomes an efficacious participation in the love, which binds Christ to the Church. Likewise, in marriage the natural attraction of man and woman is made the medium for bodily acts of love, which are genuinely sacramental.

What then is spirituality? It may be described as "'life in Christ' and 'in the Spirit,' which is accepted in faith, expressed in love and inspired by hope . . . [which] becomes the daily life of the Christian community" (John Paul II 1999, no. 29, p. 48). In other words, spirituality is the Christian life—a life comprised by the theological virtues of faith hope and love—become day-to-day praxis. Spirituality must therefore embrace all of the activities characteristic of one's vocation. In the case of marriage this includes things such as work, the preparation of meals, rest, communication, and gestures of affection—including sexual intercourse. An authentic spirituality—particularly a spirituality of marriage—must therefore embrace the body in a fundamental way. The question for this study is how NFP can contribute to such a spirituality.

Baptismal Incorporation into Christ, Marriage, and NFP

Priesthood

In the horizon of biblical thought, the body is the basis of all human relationships. It is through the body that human beings relate to the world around them, to one another, and to God (Martini 2001, 31-41). Even worship has a somatic basis, evidenced in the variety of entities from the material world offered to God in thanks, adoration, or reparation for sin. It is likewise indicated in the variety of bodily postures assumed in personal or liturgical prayer. With this background in view the Apostle Paul could exhort the Christians of Rome to offer their bodies "as a living sacrifice" (Rom. 12:1-NAB) and upbraid those in Corinth who thought nothing of engaging in ritual intercourse with a temple prostitutes for failing to consider the bodily basis of their incorporation into Christ or the dignity of their bodies as temples of the Holy Spirit (1 Cor. 6:12-20).

Biblical thought is also aware that the body's capacity for self-oblation in the worship of its Maker has an analogous representation in the self-donation of marital intercourse insofar as both are covenant-ratifying activities. Integral to the varied forms of biblical covenant is both an oath of fidelity sworn before God and some specific sign or gesture, which ratifies and recalls this oath. This latter component is generally understood as "liturgical" in nature. Thus the Israelites in concluding their pact with Yahweh at Mt. Sinai first swear faith to the terms of the covenant—"We will do everything that the Lord has told us" (Ex. 24: 3c-NAB)—then have their familial unity with Him enacted through sacrificial blood being splashed on the altar and then in turn sprinkled on them (see Ex. 24:5-8). Yet even if a covenant ratifying gesture is performed in a non-cultic setting it carries liturgical overtones, serving to both seal and recollect the faith sworn in the covenant pact. Hence the whole array of biblical gestures used in covenants may be understood in this way—a kiss, a handshake, the bestowal of gifts (Gen. 21:27; Hos. 12:2) the sharing of meals (Gen. 26:30; 31:46; Jos. 9:14-15; 2 Sam. 3:20), or the bestowal of a garment (1 Sam 18:3-4; Ez.16:8; Hugenberger 1994, 193-96, 199-200). In the case of the covenant of marriage sexual intercourse serves to both ratify and recall the oath, which the couple exchanges (Hugenberger

1994, 216-79). Like the holocaust on the altar, the bodily union of a couple serves to remember the covenant promise through a profound oblation.

Awareness of this parallel reverberates throughout the biblical and theological tradition (Grabowski 1996, 229-52). It was perhaps an inchoate understanding of the analogy between sex and worship as covenant ratifying acts that made possible the inclusion of the collection of postexilic love poetry of the Song of Songs into the canon where it was increasingly read as an allegory of divine—human love. It was on the basis of the same insight that later Christian liturgical prayers for the blessing of the nuptial chamber, such as the early medieval Spanish liturgical text, the *Liber ordinum,* named it the place of the "worthy celebration" of marriage (Searle and Stevenson 1992, 122). On similar grounds some medieval marriage liturgies, such as the thirteenth century English *Sarum Missal,* offered the following formula for the groom's gift of the ring to the bride: "With this ring, I thee wed and this gold and silver I thee give; and with my body, I thee worship, and with all my worldly chattel I thee honor" (Searle and Stevenson 1992, 167; Martinez 1988, 332-53). Such formulations are neither accidental nor aberrant. They are analogically exact ways of describing the existential intensity of the self-donation exercised by spouses both in their sexual union with one another and in their mutual worship of the Author of Love. The priesthood of the couple embraces both forms of somatic self-offering.

What has this bodily exercise of the baptismal priesthood of the couple to do with NFP? I would suggest that the use of NFP has a number of distinct and important effects on the couple in this regard. First, it produces in spouses a certain reverence for the person of the other. The study and use of the method cannot but foster in the couple a certain wonder at the intricacy of human (especially female) fertility. This wonder, coupled with the interior freedom affected by periodic continence, engenders an awareness of the other as a person—a mysterious unity of body, emotions, subjectivity, and freedom (though this is not to say that couples who do not use NFP cannot experience this wonder and reverence for the other—only that the various methods themselves foster it in specific ways). In particular, NFP enables fertility to be recognized and appreciated as a crucial element within this personal complexity and its day-to-day manifestations over time. For couples using the method to become pregnant the method makes a very practical contribution in enabling those with limited fertility to maximize its potential in becoming parents. The method thus enables husbands and wives to better perceive and treat each other as integral persons.

Second, the reverence toward one's spouse that the method imparts is manifested not only in refraining from intercourse during periods of abstinence, but by imbuing their bodily union with a heightened appreciation of their interpersonal dignity. Philosophers such as Dietrich von Hildebrand have spoken of the quality of "tenderness" that animates wedded love and makes it qualitatively different than mere "sex" (von Hildebrand 1989, 67-84). This characteristic tenderness is produced when the *intentio unitiva* on the part of the couple is adumbrated and informed by *benevolentia*. Because NFP fosters conjugal chastity through periodic continence and because it sharpens the couple's ability to perceive the totality of the other as a person it thereby enables them to promote the well-being of the other in the expression of physical love. Furthermore, the methods of expressing affection and building intimacy during periods of abstinence color a couple's sexual relationship so that it can be more clearly experienced as shared self-giving.

Third, the reverence, which the couple acquires toward one another, is an extension of the reverence toward their Creator in whose image they are created. Seeing their mutual fertility as integral to their make-up as persons, and respecting that fertility in their sexual relations so that their mutual dignity is upheld, is an expression of justice toward the God who made them (Wojtyla 1993, 245-49). This mutual reverence creates a "space" in the couple's relationship where God can be recognized as the Author of their love and the new life, which flows from it. It is little wonder that most methods of NFP insist on integrating prayer into a couple's life together as the method serves to sensitize couples to the transcendent values at stake in their sexual relationship. As such, NFP engenders a capacity in couples to offer their bodies as "spiritual sacrifices" to God in the midst of their sexual relationship with one another.

Prophecy

The human body is naturally expressive in and of itself. In its physicality and materiality it expresses or incarnates the spiritual subjectivity and freedom of the person in the world. In its visibility and concreteness it enunciates "otherness" to the personal subjects who perceive it. The most basic and primordial form of this otherness is articulated by the duality of male and female (Martini 2001, 45-50). For in sexual difference the "I" of the personal subject is formed in its self-awareness by the encounter with an irreducible "Thou." But such differences are themselves an invitation to the dialogue of friendship and mutual love. Pope John Paul II has referred to this call to communion inscribed in the fabric of personal existence as male or female as "the nuptial meaning of the body" (John Paul II 1997, weekly general audience of January 9, 1980, 60-63).

But the body speaks not only in its existence as male or female. It also speaks and expresses itself through activity. Indeed, some forms of somatic expression convey far more deeply than a multitude of words—the handshake of reconciliation between longtime enemies, the embrace of comfort given to the grieving, the caress of affection from parent to child, the kiss exchanged between lovers. Such is also the case with the bodily word of love shared by spouses in sexual intercourse. Even if no words are exchanged, this act has the ability, when rendered translucent by the medium of love and affection, to convey a gift of the whole person precisely as male or female (though it must be acknowledged that the same act, rendered opaque by resentment, frustration, or emotional withdrawal, can equally convey disdain, manipulation, or other darker utterances).

Pope John Paul II has described this somatic dialogue carried on by a married couple as "a language of the body" (John Paul II 1997, weekly general audiences of January 12 and 26, 1983, 357-60, 363-65). In his view sexual intercourse is a word rendered intelligible by the marriage covenant, which unites the couple. Within this covenantal framework, the declaration of sexual intercourse can be understood as a word of fidelity and of total self-giving. Fidelity is manifested because a couple gives themselves to one another in this way and to no other. Total self-donation because intercourse enacts in bodily form the unconditional promise and acceptance articulated by the couple in their wedding vows.

Like any language, such a word can be uttered truly or in falsehood. The married man who gives himself to another woman belies the oath of fidelity he has sworn to his wife. The couple that uses contraception contradicts the language of total self-donation uttered by their bodies (a point made repeatedly in the teaching of Pope John Paul II (*Familiaris consortio*, no. 32; *Letter to Families, Gratissimam sane*, no. 12; John Paul II 1997, weekly general audience of August 22, 1984, 396-99 Wojtyla 1993, 234). For in fact in using contraception they choose to refuse an integral part of that mutual gift bestowed on one another, i.e., their fertility. This fertility is not a disease to be medicated away or surgically removed, but a vital dimension of their make up as sexual persons. To withhold or reject it in the couple's ongoing bodily dialogue contradicts the unconditional nature of their original covenant promise. In every act of intercourse, a couple declares themselves to be not only spouses but also potential parents, collaborators with God in the creation of a new human life (John Paul II, 1997, weekly general audiences of March 12 and 26, 1980, 80-86).

Here again the contribution of NFP to marital spirituality becomes evident. For NFP assures that the word spoken by the body is spoken in truth. The couple that abstains from intercourse during fertile periods because they have good reason to avoid pregnancy utter nothing to contradict the totality of their mutual love. They simply find other ways, verbal and somatic, to convey this love, which accord with the promises they have made to one another. This is significant for a number of reasons. Ethically, it is crucial that the couple either gives themselves to one another in their personal totality or that they do not. There is no willed contradiction of the totality of this gift, which demeans one another's dignity. Psychologically, the development of means of conveying affection and love other than genital sex during periods of abstinence creates the medium in which the word of intercourse can be better perceived as a word of love. Theologically, therefore, alternation of periods of intercourse in which fertility is accepted as integral to marital self-donation with periods of abstinence serves to promote the couple's vocation to communion.

In this regard, one might speak, as Pope John Paul II has done, of the "prophetism of the body" on the part of such couples. Thus the Pope states: "On the basis of the biblical record we speak of a 'prophetism of the body.' If the human being-male and female-in marriage (and indirectly in all the spheres of mutual life together) confers on his behavior a significance in conformity with the fundamental truth of the language of the body, he also 'is in the truth'" (John Paul II 1997, weekly general audience of January 26, 1983, 363-65).

For by their use of NFP married couples fulfill their baptismal calling to announce the truth about the dignity of the human person male or female as an integral whole. They affirm the goodness of the body, the holiness of marriage, and the beauty of sexual intercourse which preserves its meaning as total self-donation. At the same time, they take a prophetic stand against the reduction of sex to mere pleasure or techné within the culture in which they live. And they eschew the point of view that sees fertility as a disease and an obstacle to sexual flourishing rather than a gift and blessing from God. In this way, such couples give a witness that is both practical and prophetic and allow their day-to-day lives to be permeated with the light of gospel.

Kingship

From its beginning, Christianity has insisted that authority is not to be used for the acquisition of power and privilege, but rather for the sake of service. This insistence was based on the example of Jesus himself who the Gospels state came not "to be served but to serve and to give his life as a ransom for many" (Mk.10:45-NAB). This conviction explains the ancient Christian axiom "to serve is to reign." Christians who are therefore baptized into Christ and anointed with his royal chrism are initiated into a life of service.

This has immediate implications for men and women who are united in marriage and who have children. Relatively early on the Christian East developed the practice of placing crowns on the heads of newly married couples when they received the Eucharist for the first time as a couple (Olsen, 2001,115; Roth 1986, 12-14). This liturgical gesture signifies the restoration of the royal dignity of Adam and Eve made present again in creation in the persons of this couple (Evdokimov 1995, 148-56). But this act acknowledges their royal dignity is simultaneously a summons to a life of mutual service. Most of the day-to-day activities of a family can be understood as expressions of such service: the preparation of food; the cleaning of the home; caring for sick members of the family; nurturing the unborn, the young or the elderly; welcoming others into the home in hospitality; or action outside of the home to promote greater solidarity with the poor and disadvantaged (Parella 1982, 139-41).

It is not accidental that again the body is the locus of these expressions of Christian kingship. Jesus himself insisted that his disciples encountered him in the bodily care of those hungry, thirsty, naked, ill, or imprisoned (Matt. 25: 31-46). He likewise demonstrated his own care of his followers by performing the office of a servant and washing their feet (Jn. 13:1-17). Christian preachers and mystics throughout history have kept alive this insight by directing other believers to find their Lord in the persons of the marginalized—to use Mother Theresa's prophetic words "in the poorest of the poor."

The body is not only the basis of the person's ability to offer him or herself in love or to speak this word in love and truth, it is the basis of human vulnerability, weakness, and need. The Hebrew *basar,* which can be rendered 'flesh' or 'body,' has a whole array of these associations. "All flesh is grass" (Is. 40:6) the prophet acknowledges in the face of the reality of human weakness and mortality (KJV—while many modern translations render the Hebrew as "mankind" [NAB] or "all men" [NIV], in this case the poetic rendering of the King James is also a more literal translation of *basar).*

The vulnerability of the body is also acknowledged in the very act of marrying. In Genesis, the man awakens from his covenant sleep and declares, "this one at last is bone of my bone and flesh of my flesh." Scholars have pointed out that bone is a symbol of strength and solidity in biblical thought while flesh denotes its opposite (Bruggeman 1970, 532-42). The couple in more contemporary wedding vows embraces the same range of human possibility when they bind themselves to each other "in sickness and in health." Thus part of a couple's vocation is to learn to serve one another in day-to-day acts of bodily care, especially during periods of vulnerability or illness. This body-induced range of possibilities has obvious implications for a couple's sexual relationship as it flows directly from the health

NFP & Marital Spirituality

and vitality of the couple. The sexual relationship of a young newly married couple will be rather different than an elderly couple struggling with poor health. Yet, it may well be that the love, affection, and tenderness expressed in this latter relationship is far greater than that between the newlyweds.

What bearing does NFP have on the capacity of a married couple to live their vocation to "wash one another's feet" through daily service? It is fairly obvious that the practice of periodic continence at various points in their relationship better prepares couples for those times when due to childbirth, illness, or advanced age they are unable to engage in intercourse. The couple that has developed an array of non-genital means to express love and affection will be able to share such periods with greater serenity. Daily physical acts of care from sharing a walk together, to holding hands, to giving a foot rub, to helping a spouse to wash and dress during an illness are embodied acts of nuptial kingship. Such acts will not be foreign to those accustomed to expressing love within the periodic continence of NFP.

Less obvious is the way in which the use of NFP nudges the couple to deeper communication and mutuality in their daily service of one another. The method directs the couple to attend to their shared fertility and to discuss it in the context of their overall relationship. Given the intensely personal nature of sexuality, even some married couples hesitate to discuss their sexual relationship with one another. NFP builds a praxis of mutual communication which in turn makes it more difficult for a spouse to look at their sexual relationship from the vantage of only his or her own needs—and therefore makes this relationship less subject to univocal demands, manipulation, or power statements. NFP therefore helps to integrate the language of the body into the daily fabric of mutual love and service.

This communication in turn produces a deeper mutuality in the life of the couple. NFP impels them to make decisions about intercourse and pregnancy together. This mutuality in the area of decisions about sex creates a momentum within the life of the couple to operate in similar fashion elsewhere in the relationship—in decisions about raising children, finances, and the practice of their faith. The method thereby accords with the New Testament injunction recently highlighted by the Church for couples to "be subordinate to one another out of reverence for Christ" (Eph. 5:21-NAB) in their lives of sacrificial service and mutual deference (see 5:22-33; *Mulieris dignitatem*, no. 24 in John Paul II 1997, 478-479).

Conclusion:
Toward a Spirituality of Marital Sexuality

The theory and praxis of NFP makes a contribution to an authentic spirituality of marriage because it takes the body seriously. Unlike previous approaches to marital spirituality which tended to ignore the body as male or female in the spiritual life or at least to minimize its place therein, NFP resists these efforts. For the method begins with the body. It takes the body and its fertility as givens and as good and seeks to integrate them into the whole fabric of the couple's life and relationship. But the method also resists a materialist view of the person for it sees the body and its capacity for love, self-donation, and parenthood as pointing beyond itself to the transcendent values at stake in human sexuality. In respecting one another as integral persons, the couple acknowledges that it is ultimately God who is the source and goal of their love and the author of the new life, which flows from it.

This is not to say that the use of NFP constitutes the whole of a spirituality of marriage. A couple's sexual relationship is only a small—though vital—part of their overall life together. Spirituality must embrace the whole of that life. In this regard, it is instructive to consider the way in which John Paul II has suggested that the "language of the body" spoken by the couple can be understood to encompass all the words, gestures, and moments of their history together as their mutual attraction matures through the Holy Spirit's work of deepening their reverence for one another (1 Thes. 4:4-7; John Paul II 1997, weekly general audience of July 4, 1984, 378-80).

But NFP, particularly its practice, can make a real contribution to the overall spiritual life and growth of couples. Its use helps them to find in their bodily offering of themselves to one another a growing reverence for one another's dignity as persons, which is an extension and manifestation of their reverence for their Creator. It enables them to speak this bodily word of love to one another in truth and in the context of a relationship in which intimacy is fostered in a variety of ways. And it assists them in integrating this dialogue into a life of mutual service, communication, and shared authority. For these reasons the use of NFP can assist couples in living their baptismal incorporation into Christ and their marital consecration to holiness.

In thus helping to reconnect marital spirituality with marital sexuality, the theory and practice of NFP serves to model an integrated and healthy understanding of sexuality within the Church and the broader culture. For NFP promotes an understanding of sex that locates it within the covenantal union of a man and a woman who relate to one another as whole persons called together in love. As such it stands in opposition to the many manic expressions of sex within the contemporary world which sees it as nothing more than a commodity to be consumed, the search for happiness truncated to mere pleasure, the calculated negation of total self-donation, or the expression of control in the name of misguided love, i.e., pornography, casual sex, contraceptive sex, or sexual abuse of those who are vulnerable due to age or position. The theory and practice of NFP helps us to perceive what sane sex is and can be according to the Creator's design. As such, it points toward a spirituality, which affirms with St. Irenaeus that the glory of God is the human person fully alive (*Adversus haereses* 4, 20, 7).

Bibliography

Abbott, S.J., Walter. Ed. 1966. *The Documents of Vatican II*. Piscataway, NJ: New Century Publishers.

Augustine, Saint. *De bono conjugali* (*The Good of Marriage*). In Defarrari, Roy J. Ed. 1955. *The Fathers of the Church*. Vol. 27, translated by Charles T. Wilcox *et al*, 9-51. Washington, D.C.: The Catholic University of America Press.

Bruggeman, S.J. Walter. 1970. "Of the Same Flesh and Bone." *Catholic Biblical Quarterly* 32: 532-42.

dos Anjos, Márcio Fabri. 1995. "Building a Spirituality of Family Life." In Cahill, Lisa Sowle & Mieth, Dietmar. Eds. *Concilium, The Family* 4: 99-109.

Elliott, Dyan. 1993. *Spiritual Marriage: Sexual Abstinence in Medieval Wedlock*. Princeton, N.J.: Princeton University Press.

Evdokimov, Paul. 1995. *The Sacrament of Love*. Translated by. Anthony Gythiel and Victoria Steadman. Crestwood, N.Y.: St. Vladimir's Seminary Press.

Grabowski, John S. 1996. "Covenantal Sexuality." *Église et Théologie* 27: 229-52.

———. 1997. "Mutual Submission and Trinitarian Self-Giving." *Angelicum* 74: 489-512.

Hugenberger, Gordon Paul. 1994. *Marriage as a Covenant: A Study of Biblical Law and Ethics Developed from the Perspective of Malachi.* Supplements to Vetus Testamentum. Leiden: Brill, 52.

John Paul II. 1988. *Christifideles laici.* Apostolic Exhortation. Liberia Editrice Vaticana translation. Washington, D.C.: United State Catholic Conference.

———. 1997. *The Theology of the Body: Human Love in the Divine Plan.* Translated by *L'Osservatore Romano*, English Edition. Boston: Pauline Books and Media.

———. 1999. *Ecclesia in America.* Apostolic Exhortation. Liberia Editrice Vaticana translation. Washington, D.C.: United States Catholic Conference.

Mahoney, S.J., John. 1987. *The Making of Moral Theology: A Study of the Roman Catholic Tradition.* Oxford: Clarendon.

Martinez, Germán. 1988. "Marriage as Worship: A Theological Analogy." *Worship* 62: 332-53.

Martini, Carlo Maria. 2001. *On the Body: A Contemporary Theology of the Human Person.* Translated by Rosanna M. Giammanco Frongia. New York: Crossroad.

Olsen, Glenn W. 2001. "Progeny, Faithfulness, Sacred Bond: Marriage in the Age of Augustine." In Olsen, Glenn. Ed. *Christian Marriage: A Historical Study.* New York: Herder and Herder, 101-45.

Örsy, S.J.,Ladislas. 1997. "Married People: God's Chosen People." In Demmer, Klaus & Brenninkmeijer-Werhahn, Aldegonde. Eds. *Christian Marriage Today.* Washington, D.C.: Catholic University of America Press, 38-54.

Parrella, Frederick J. 1982. "Towards a Spirituality of the Family." *Communio.* 9: 127-41.

Rochetta, Carlo. 1997. "Marriage as a Sacrament: Toward a New Theological Conceptualization." In Demmer, Klaus & Brenninkmeijer-Werhahn, Aldegonde. Eds. *Christian Marriage Today.* Washington, D.C.: Catholic University of America Press, 55-80.

Roth, Catherine P. 1986. Introduction to *On Marriage and Family Life*, by Saint John Chrysostom. Translated by Catherine P. Roth and David Anderson. Crestwood, N.Y.: St. Vladimir's Seminary.

Von Hildebrand, Dietrich. 1931. *In Defense of Purity.* Reprint *Purity: The Mystery of Christian Sexuality.* Steubenville, OH: Franciscan University Press, 1989.

Wojtyla, Karol. 1981. *Love and Responsibility.* Translated by H.T. Willets. New York: Farrar, Straus and Giroux. Reprint San Francisco: Ignatius, 1993.

Response to John Grabowski

John Grabowski's paper is a ray of sunlight that pierces through the overcast skies under which we Catholics have lived of late. Although he wrote the paper at something of a theoretical level—in other words, he was not intent upon being a commentator on current events—the fact is that what he has to say is applicable to current events, to our contemporary culture. With perspectives garnered from Dr. Grabowski's paper, I would like to tease out some applications of his efforts.

Like other appetites that work to sustain the life of the individual or the life of the species, the human sexual appetite has a tendency to consume one's thoughts, rather than to moderate them. Since we rarely encounter people who suffer from the vice of insensitivity (wanting sex too little), but rather more often encounter people who suffer from an excessive desire for sexual activity, it comes as no surprise that traditionally the way to deal with the allure of sexuality is to put it away altogether (Aristotle claims that, to begin working away on a vice, we often have to go to its opposite extreme). Hence the emphasis upon the virgin or celibate life in Christian monastic tradition, and in Christian theology generally. St. Augustine's teaching that celibacy is inherently preferable to marriage is sometimes thought to be an overreaction on his part to his own, sexually care-free, youth.

Whatever the precise causes of our theological tradition's handling of marital, or sexual, spirituality, Dr. Grabowski's paper provides married persons with an idea of how their particular vocation—which alone legitimately includes sexual activity—is a distinctive participation in the Lord's mission. Married people, in a married way, are to be priests, prophets, and kings, just as the Lord, in a more universal way—and perhaps because of his celibacy—was a priest, prophet, and king, all the way to Calvary.

So every Christian is part of the priesthood of all believers, and therefore exercises the functions of priesthood, prophecy, and kingship, in the vocation to which he or she is eventually called—the ordained priest at the altar and in the confessional, the monk in a cloister, members of religious orders in ways according to their charasm, the consecrated single person in his or her way. Yet there remains one way of life that all share in at some point in their life: living in the world, *in seculo*, which is the precise provenance of marriage. That is to say that everyone, being born into a family of some kind, spends at least some time or even a long time—an entire childhood, perhaps—"in the world," even before the options of becoming a priest or entering a convent or monastery offer themselves.

As Dr. Grabowski notes, citing Vatican II's *Lumen gentium*, the laity are characterized by "secularity," that is, by living in this world. And thus the married Catholic is "in this world," though not necessarily "of this world"—and that distinction is important, now more than ever. For, it is the married Catholic, employing theoretic considerations of marital spirituality like those just offered by Dr. Grabowksi, and personally aware of the reality of human sexuality, who can navigate in a world he or she knows with a message that the world does not know, but needs to know: that sex can be not only part of a holy life, but a holy part of a holy life. As you may know, the English term 'holy,' meaning 'sacred,' and 'whole,' meaning 'complete' or 'entire' or 'intact,' are related, and Dr. Grabowski notes how the married couple respects the entirety of each other in the practice of NFP, neither elevating nor minimizing either the physical or the spiritual element of the other spouse to the point of exclusion of the other. In fact, apart from the somewhat immediate goal of avoiding pregnancy in cases of serious necessity or of becoming pregnant when a child is sought, it might be said that the principal accomplishment of NFP is the integration of the physical and the spiritual in human nature, driven by the belief in the divine wisdom, who made us to be this way. The couple practicing NFP therefore begins their thinking with the contention that we are not so much makers of ourselves as we are receivers of ourselves, receiving our very natures from God. That thinking, when applied in the manner Dr. Grabowksi presents, is holy because it does justice to God's handiwork, our very human selves.

Since everyone spends at least some time "in the world," and in our case as parents, it is crucial to take that opportunity to teach by word and deed what true sexuality is, for the pressures and orthodoxies of the world quickly set upon the young with promises of instant joy, where true love demands patience, total autonomy, where genuine fulfillment requires service to others. If there is one thing that I would dare add to Dr. Grabowksi's paper, it is the somewhat odd request that NFP-practicing couples let everyone see them being sexual—"sexual," that is, in the Christ-like way they live their married lives as sexual beings, not being afraid to bear prophetic witness to the truth of NFP by living their integrated lives publicly, in the world. Live vibrantly, live proud, live sexy. Sex is a joy for us just as much as it is a joy for the world. But we, being in the world but not of the world, know that sex is but a single joy among many—it is not all our joy, and is still less the greatest joy. Sex is a joy that, in truth, pales in comparison to those promised us by Christ our King. We thank Dr. Grabowksi for so clearly spelling all this out.

Mark F. Johnson, Ph.D.
Associate Professor
Department of Theology
Marquette University

Contraception, Natural Family Planning, and Women

Teresa Wagner, Esq.
Washington, DC

Introduction

I began to appreciate the Church's teachings on human sexuality when my husband-to-be and I took part in a week-long seminar called the "Fundamentals of the Faith," sponsored by the Withersfield Institute at Notre Dame University. During that week, Professor Janet Smith helped participants better understand the Church's teaching on contraception. Of course, the Church's insight in this area is not reserved for Catholic couples; it can assist anyone hoping to understand human sexuality and its connection to human dignity and human life. For that reason, I try to pass along the Church's insights whenever it is appropriate to do so.

I was disappointed, therefore, when a fellow orthodox Catholic friend (who agrees with the Church's teaching) suggested that the Church "give up" on contraception. My reaction: We can't give up on something we haven't even tried. But two other thoughts quickly followed: First, contraception is the basis of several destabilizing developments in our culture over the past 40 years, including sex before marriage, general promiscuity, out-of-wedlock pregnancy, abortion, illegitimacy, adultery and divorce. The total separation of sex from children also leads to human manipulations, such as human cloning and embryonic stem cell research. "Give up" on this issue? Only if we are prepared to live with such de-stabilizing results, past, present and future.

Second, a review of recent public policy initiatives shows a tendency on the part of those who support contraception and abortion to press for more than legalization and tolerance. They really want *endorsement*, but as they work to achieve this, they lobby for support—financial, social and political—and are ready to coerce such support against the wills and consciences of others.

For example, many laws now require not only that state health insurance plans (taxpayer-subsidized) pay for contraceptive drugs and devices, but also that private employer plans do the same—including insurance plans provided by the Catholic Church for its employees.

These destabilizing and coercive trends can be expected to continue and expand. When human sexuality is divorced from "having children," such practices follow as a matter of logic, as do their legal mandates. The connection between sex and children, or between life and love, which is the heart of the Church's teaching on contraception, turns out to be a linchpin.

In this presentation I will discuss various public policy measures on mandatory contraception coverage. Second, I will compare contraception to Natural Family Planning from the perspective of *female appreciation*. And finally, I will discuss our contraceptive culture, which does not understand or appreciate female fertility, and how it can foster hostile attitudes toward women, children and families.

1. Contraception in Law & Public Policy

The most active front for contraception promotion is the campaign to mandate contraceptive coverage as part of health insurance plans. At present, most traditional indemnity plans (fee-for-service insurance), preferred provider plans (PPOs) and health maintenance organizations (HMOs) do not include contraceptives as a "health benefit." Instead, individuals purchase contraceptives with their own money.

Businesses give various reasons for this. The Chamber of Commerce, for example, cites costs, as well as the need for employer discretion in tailoring packages for employees (Sullivan 2001). Contraceptive advocates, unhappy with this situation, have been trying for years to have the law require businesses to include contraception in their health benefits packages. Contraception advocates call this "equity" or "parity" for women in medical coverage, and their efforts have met with considerable success.

One important note: Many people refer to contraception as a "health benefit," or as satisfying a "basic health need" in this debate. Indeed, Senator Barbara Mikulski (D-Md.), a leader in the campaign to mandate contraceptive coverage, calls contraception a "medical necessity" (Id.). The first "talking point" for those who advocate mandated contraception is, "Contraception is *basic health care* for women." It doesn't hurt their cause that contraception has all the trappings of medicine – drug stores, prescriptions, doctor visits, etc., As a result, those who oppose such mandates are seen as trying to deprive others of a "benefit" or "basic need," already a disadvantage in terms of public perception. Few challenge the terminology since few are willing to explain that *human fertility* is actually healthy.

Advocates of mandated contraceptive coverage have met with alarming success. For example:

Legislation: Federal Level

A. Federal Employee Health Benefits Program (FEHBP)

FEHBP is the health insurance plan for federal government employees. Accordingly, it is the largest employer-sponsored health plan in the world, with some nine million enrollees. It is paid for by all tax-paying Americans. In 1998, Congress made contraceptives a "health benefit" under this plan (effective 1999).

B. Equity in Prescription Insurance and Contraceptive Coverage Bill

Originally introduced to Congress in 1997, the Equity in Prescription Insurance and Contraceptive Coverage bill or EPICC bill, has been reintroduced each year without passing. This bill, and similar bills and laws in several states, would require any health plan providing prescription drugs and devices, as well as medical outpatient services, to include all FDA-approved contraceptive drugs, devices or outpatient "services." It forbids penalties or limits on reimbursements for those who prescribe or administer contraception, and allows such products to be subject to deductibles and co-payments, provided other prescriptions are similarly treated. Experimental contraceptives must be covered if other experimental prescription drugs are covered. In short, contraceptives are to be treated like any other FDA-approved medicines.

One should also note the importance of FDA approval in the federal language. Although this paper is not about the possible abortifacient nature of certain drugs and devices that are marketed as contraceptives, one can see how normalization of contraception also plays into the hands of abortion advocates. Despite a *de facto* policy of legal abortion throughout pregnancy, abortion remains controversial in the U.S., much to the dismay of its advocates. This is not so with contraception, which, by some estimates is used by 80% of adult Americans (Critchlow 1999). Categorizing abortion-inducing drugs as contraceptives can therefore help normalize abortion in public policy. For example, a 1998 letter from the Office of Personal Management (OPM), the federal agency which administers the insurance program, states that plans participating in FEHBP must offer the "full range of contraceptive drugs and devices approved for use by the Food and Drug Administration." This list includes the IUD and the morning after pill, both of which can cause abortion. In effect, federal policy approves of and pays for early abortion, since drugs with this capability are offered as health benefits under the FEHBP. Not only does this run counter to current federal policy on funding for abortion (that is, the Hyde Amendment), it has consequences for the status of the human embryo in other areas of federal law, such as fetal experimentation or embryonic stem cell research.

During Senate Hearings in 2001, only one person - a representative of the U.S. Chamber of Commerce - testified against the pending bill on the grounds that mandated coverage would "further increase costs" of health care, and thus would "jeopardize the affordability and availability of health plans for workers." Such cost-benefit analyses hardly move the human heart. What's more, most people only see that contraception is less costly than abortion, and certainly less costly than pregnancy and childbirth. So this line of argument will not get the Chamber very far. Policies promoting chastity on the other hand–both before and during marriage–would be most cost effective of all. But this option is not even entertained.

Legislation: State Level

Since 1998, twenty states have passed laws comparable to the federal EPPC bill. Maryland was the first state to do so in 1998, followed by California, Connecticut, Georgia, Hawaii, Maine, Nevada, New Hampshire in 1999. Delaware, Iowa and Rhode Island passed laws in 2000. Missouri, New Mexico, Texas, Washington, North Carolina and Vermont did so in 2001, and in 2002, Massachusetts, Arizona, and New York passed such laws. This is quite a record in less than four years.

Litigation

Along with the effort to enact federal and state laws is a litigation strategy—suing employers on the basis of sex discrimination when their health plans do not cover contraception. This strategy has also met with considerable success. In December of 2000, for example, the Equal Employment Opportunity Commission ruled that any health plan covering preventive services, but not prescription contraceptives, discriminated on the basis of sex, in violation of the Civil Rights Act of 1964 and the Pregnancy Discrimination Act. Although significant, this decision was an administrative agency ruling, which lacks the import of court precedent. But less than a year later such a court decision came down in the case of *Erickson v. Bartell Drug Company* (144 F. Supp, 2d 1266 2001).

Erickson, which received enormous media attention, involved a female pharmacist (Jennifer Erickson) who sued her employer, Bartell Drug Company, claiming that Bartell's exclusion of contraception in its health plan (the firm is self-insured) constituted sex discrimination under Title VII of the 1964 Civil Rights Act. In June 2001, the federal district court in Seattle agreed. Title VII prohibits an employer from discriminating against an individual on the basis of race, religion, color, sex or national origin. A prospective employer cannot discriminate in hiring or compensation practices, and health benefit plans have been interpreted as part of compensation. The Court found that sex-based differences between men and women sometimes require employers to provide women-only benefits and/or otherwise incur additional expenses on behalf of women, in order to treat the sexes equally. Simply put, employers must sometimes treat men and women differently in order to treat them equally since men and women have different needs especially in the area of healthcare. (The Court was actually interpreting the 1979 amendment to Title VII, called the Pregnancy Discrimination Act.)

This principle is sound as far as it goes. Men and women are different and sometimes warrant different treatment. The problem is not the principle or the reasoning of the Court, or even the reasoning of the advocates before it. The problem is accepting contraception as healthcare in the first place! It is not. But once you have accepted this, it is entirely foreseeable and logical that efforts to expand medical coverage will include efforts to promote contraception.

In defending itself, Bartell argued:

1. Contraception is different from other prescription drugs, in that they do not treat or prevent disease and therefore are *not truly health care*;
2. Control of fertility is not used in the language of the 1979 Pregnancy Discrimination Act;
3. Employers must have discretion in formulating packages in order to control costs;
4. Bartell excludes *all* family planning drugs (including infertility treatments) so contraception exclusion is neutral, not discriminatory;
5. No court has ever before required an employer to cover contraception;
6. This issue is fundamentally a policy decision for legislators to make, not the courts.

All these points are valid, but the first goes to the heart of the matter: Contraceptives do not prevent disease and are not truly health care.

Public Policy Issues

The biggest issue surrounding contraception mandates is conscience protection for those who object to contraceptive use. Contraception advocates lobby for absolute mandates, or failing that, very narrow protection for those with religious objections; they reject protection for those with moral objections (objections not grounded in any specific religious tenet). For example, when this issue was raised in 2002 with the D.C. appropriations bill in Congress, many on the D.C. City Council lobbied Congress not only to narrow conscience protection for those with objections, but to make organizations pay the costs of verification (to ensure that the organizations were sufficiently religious to qualify for the exemption). As the U.S. Bishops' Conference said at the time, such narrowing efforts, coupled with levying fines, are not genuine conscience protection. I would add that such "narrowing efforts" are the beginning of state coercion. In the end, the FEHPB mandate protected religious *and moral* objections of individual health care providers, but only the religious objections of health care *plans*.

A Feminist Perspective of NFP & Contraception

Commentary – Conscience Clause Protection

The issue of conscience protection, however, skips over *the* most important matter here—whether contraception is healthcare at all, and whether its widespread use is good health care and social policy.

It is true that such mandates violate individual consciences, as well as Church teaching since they force individual Catholics, and others, to pay premiums for contraceptive drugs and devices. And we certainly need to protect against such violations.

What's more, if the law declares contraception a benefit all must subsidize, then the law—by logic and principle—can compel fuller participation: e.g., physical assistance (filling prescriptions, distributing drugs and devices), contribution of expertise (research and development within the pharmaceutical industry) and advice (counseling women on how to administer contraceptives), etc. The groundwork for more material cooperation has been laid.

Thus, resistance to mandatory contraception coverage by the Church and others is well-founded. Indeed, the main problem is that this resistance is so narrow-cast (only the Catholic Church has been visibly in opposition) and not well developed (the reasons for opposition to contraception are rarely explained). The focus is almost exclusively on respect for conscientious objection.

Commentary—the Morality of Contraception

I would like to look now at the need to explain the Church's position.

The Catholic Church has steadfastly maintained a teaching against artificial contraception. Yet often it seems to do so without confidence, and perhaps even with some embarrassment. There may be many reasons for this. For example, human sexuality is profoundly mysterious and intimate. Discomfort may well be a sign of respect for its power and mystery. Whatever the reasons, the result has been a failure to teach and lead, creating a vacuum that popular culture, with its denigration of sex, has filled. This, in turn, has been a great deprivation for the faithful. There are many Catholics who do not understand and thus cannot appreciate the Church's insight into human sexuality and how necessary these truths are to human dignity and the protection of human life.

One can understand why the Church works to exempt itself from contraception mandates. Such defensive moves are natural and may suffice to protect the Church today. But in the meantime, acceptance of contraception by the medical and business communities legitimizes contraception for everyone else. Without instruction from the Church, people of other faiths wonder why Catholics maintain this "quirky" position, even as society moves toward more and more sexual promiscuity and degradation. A teaching moment is lost, as they say. Worse still, Catholics themselves begin to accept contraception because everyone else does, and because the Church has not provided compelling reasons to avoid it.

So tomorrow, when the Church works to exempt itself from yet another mandate, its position is weaker. Why should the Church be an exception when its own people want contraception as a covered benefit? Since time has passed without explanation of why contraception is not a "good," many simply see an inequity in contraception exclusion – including our courts.

We cannot continue to evade the issue. The Church must explain its teaching or risk being co-opted by a contraceptive culture that gives lip service to respect for human sexuality and human life itself.

2. Fertility Versus Infertility: Which Constitutes Health?

Over the past ten years, there has also been a parallel effort to mandate *in*fertility treatment. Here might be an opportune moment for the Church and Natural Family Planning advocates. Infertility as a medical problem is instructive. It raises a very fundamental question that people fail to ask: Which condition warrants medical attention? Fertility or infertility?

It seems to me you can't have it both ways. Either the ability to conceive (fertility) is a healthy condition, and the inability to conceive (infertility) merits medical attention; or the ability to conceive requires medical correction (the contraceptive pill) and infertility is a good. Which is it?

For the modern mindset neither is true. Or both are true – since reality is nothing other than what one wants. If you choose to have sex and do not want children, fertility is the problem and the medical profession should *fix* it. If you choose to have sex and *do* want children,

A Feminist Perspective of NFP & Contraception

infertility is the problem and the medical profession should fix it. The only relevant factor is what one wants. This viewpoint ignores a natural order, because human beings *appear* able to successfully manipulate, dominate, or control certain natural processes, and so "human will" is all that matters.

Such manipulations, if not a cooperation with nature, will exact a price. Humans cannot dominate and manipulate nature to their own ends without a fall-out because nature has a balance and an order of its own that must be accommodated. The modern mind seems totally oblivious to the natural order as an objective reality that needs to be understood and respected. As Pope Paul VI points out in *Humanae vitae*:

> [M]an has made stupendous progress in the domination and rational organization of the forces of nature, such that he tends to extend this domination to his own total being: to the body, to psychical life, to social life and even to the laws which regulate the transmission of life. (#2)

But this viewpoint can never trump in the field of medicine. Doctors study the human body first – they learn its parts and functions and how it reacts to outside forces. They understand the concept of what is healthy (when the body is doing what it should, all parts are functioning as intended) and not healthy (when the body is not doing what it should). Only with this foundation can the art of medicine truly develop.

In other words, ideologues can be enamored of choice to the point of ignoring the reality of the human body and what is healthy. Doctors can not do this because medicine is the cooperation of humans and nature: humans helping the body do what it was made to do.

Fertility as a Condition of Health

Though simplistic, the question also points to a fundamental truth that informs Catholic doctrine: The woman who can conceive (get pregnant and carry a child) is *healthy*. Her body is doing what it is *supposed* to do, what it was created to do. It follows that the woman (or the couple) who cannot easily conceive may need medical attention because something is *not* functioning correctly.

Sadly, the medical profession takes a pass on this question, inviting an entire industry to develop drugs and devices unique to the medical world, because they alter a perfectly healthy condition – the natural condition of fertility. But precisely because contraceptive drugs and devices do not restore health or correct a deficiency, they are not, properly speaking, medical services, despite their medical trappings.

Fertility Awareness as Appreciation of the Female: Manipulation or Respect?

Since human fertility is based on female fertility (the male is constantly fertile; the female is cyclically fertile), the push to simply control fertility meant a lost opportunity to learn about and in turn respect, the woman's role in human reproduction. On this point, we should be clear that NFP is not only a form of fertility awareness, but fertility *appreciation* and specifically, appreciation of *female* fertility (ultimately, appreciation of the woman*)*. While no person can be reduced to his or her physical attributes, fertility cycles are indisputably feminine. How we treat this cycle tells us something about our attitude toward women.

Proponents of contraception, intent on being able to control and manipulate fertility, are oblivious to the sophisticated and delicate ecology of the human female. Thus the first obvious difference between contraception use and NFP is this: The former manipulates the female body and therefore never learns to respect it or women generally; the latter requires understanding of the female fertility cycle, fosters respect for it and for women generally.

Gift or Nuisance?

What's more, NFP actually has an entirely different view of human sexuality. NFP teaches that sex is a sacred gift. It is an expression of love and the source of life, the impulse of giving and creating. It is the human being's moment to cooperate with God in bringing into being a new human. *Humanae vitae* translations refer to the "mission" or "duty" to transmit life, which sounds rather technical. But the essence of the teaching, as far as I can tell, is that not only is each human being made in the image of God and therefore sacred, but that the means to bring human beings into existence are also sacred.

A Feminist Perspective of NFP & Contraception 59

And just as each child is a new and wondrous gift of God, so too is human sexuality, which allows for each child's creation.

Given this, manipulations of human fertility (of what is already healthy) are not to be taken lightly. Again, to quote *Humanae vitae*:

> [Man] has no such dominion over his generative faculties as such, because of their intrinsic ordination towards raising up life, of which God is the principle. "Human life is sacred," Pope John XXIII recalled; "from its very inception, it reveals the creating hand of God." (#13)

While analogies are obviously limited in accuracy and usefulness, I have in the past likened human fertility to a musical gift – since we speak about someone being "gifted" in the area of musical ability. When one sings beautifully, we say she has a great gift. Now if a singer smoked, did drugs, or drank alcohol to excess because it was "fun" or "felt good" to do so, and his voice was gradually destroyed, people would be puzzled. One expects a singer to take care, even treasure, such a gift.

Contraceptive use, far from seeing human sexuality as a gift, sees it as a nuisance that we should alter and control. Why a nuisance? Because of children. By definition, contraception is against conception—against children. As indicated earlier, human sexuality is in part sacred because it is the means by which we bring a person into the world. When a society attempts to remove children from human sexuality, it cannot but denigrate human sexuality.

This is not to say that sex without children, the infertile married couple) is degrading or immoral. However, to consciously remove children from sex is to remove an integral part of a system which is not only healthy and whole, in a medical sense, but good and holy in a religious one.

In defending conjugal morals in their integral wholeness . . . (*Humanae vitae*, #18)

One last item: Who or what really controls with the practice of contraception? Does the woman control, or do contraceptive chemicals and devices? This seems to me to be an important question. Often we hear of the importance of independence when what is really meant is a shift of dependence from one area to another. Those who speak on behalf of "feminist" organizations are horrified by a woman's dependence on her husband, for example. But these same feminists approve of dependence on government. Promotion of contraception is basically the illusion of control and independence because (a) women typically become *dependent* on drugs or contraceptive devices, rather than working with, or relying on, nature or God; and (b) these drugs and devices do not always do what they promise to do, as the high incidence of abortion among contracepting couples attests.

Contraception as anti-woman

Interestingly, most fertility manipulations have been geared toward women, with the sole exception of the condom. As far as invasive drugs and devices go, all are made for and marketed to women, with the sales pitch of "control."

Now, if fertility is correctly associated with women, and society embraces anti-fertility attitudes to the point that contraception is deemed a "right," a "benefit," even a "necessity." How pro-woman is that? Not very!

No human being should ever be reduced to his or her physical attributes. But the ability to conceive and bear children *is* uniquely feminine. When society views fertility as bothersome, or something that needs to be fixed, this easily translates into society's view of women – that *they* are a nuisance, that medicine should fix *them*, that they should be controlled or manipulated. This is simply the flip side of the point made earlier that NFP is not just fertility awareness but fertility *appreciation*, and an opportunity to respect not just the female cycle, in all its sophistication, but to appreciate women in general.

It is a great irony that women have been so easily convinced that invasive, anti-fertility drugs and devices are good for them. While the desire to space children, or limit family size, is understandable and part of responsible family planning, the acceptance of products which work against the female body, and therefore against women, should not be .

Bibliography

Critchlow, Donald T. 1999. *Intended Consequences: Birth Control, Abortion, and the Federal Government in Modern America.* New York: Oxford University Press.

Paul VI. 1968. *Humanae Vitae.* Papal Encyclical. Boston: St. Paul Books.

Sullivan, Kate. September 10, 2001. *Testimony of Kate Sullivan, Director of Health Care Policy, U.S. Chamber of Commerce. Hearing before Senate Committee on Health, Education, Labor, and Pensions.*

Erickson v. Bartell Drug Company, 144 F. Supp. 2d 1266 (W.D. Wash 2001).

Response to Theresa Wagner, Esq.

I come from a family with a history of activism. My grandmother was in the forefront of teaching the disabled. Her daughter, my mother, told her minister that if she had to say the word "obey" in her wedding vows, she would not be married. When the open housing marches occurred in Milwaukee in the 1960s, she was right there. My mother's FBI file was a source of pride in my family.

So when I announced that I was going to be a doctor, I was supported, guarded though it was. At the time, being a doctor was not something little girls dreamed about, especially if they wanted to get married and have a family. When one of my relatives asked me what I was going to be when I "grew up," she didn't believe me. "Nah," she said. "Only boys can be doctors." But I told her that girls could be doctors and I was going to be one.

I was able to go to medical school because of the women's movement. Until about a year before I entered Loyola-Stritch School of Medicine, there was one or two women, usually a nun, in a sea of male faces. Male students complained that female students were taking the place of men who would work longer hours. A surgeon once told me that I was not a real doctor because I was a woman!

Even as a resident, when I was pregnant, I was called on the carpet because I carried a bag of popcorn to settle my stomach. It was unprofessional. No one bothered to observe that it was more unprofessional to vomit on patients. And while practicing medicine, I actually got a ticket once for parking in the doctor's parking lot! But slowly women in medicine began to be treated differently. Today doctors, both women and men, are considered equally competent.

I remind you of all this because sometimes we forget the needed reforms that the women's movement initially made. But sadly, there are so many things that the women's movement failed to improve, and in fact, have even worsened—our most fundamental roles as wives and mothers. That troubles me greatly.

Today, women in traditionally "male professions" are respected. It is easier to get into them; however female professions are still considered of lower status (and often come with lower pay). Nursing is perhaps

Response to Wagner

one exception. The lowest profession of all is, of course, motherhood. Feminists look down on it more than any man ever would. Even child care workers are at the lower level of the totem pole.

The women's movement has not improved male/female relationships—they are not more stable today than in the past. As a child, I had heard that men could "get away" with abandoning their wives and children; women could not. Instead of demanding more accountability from men, the women's movement supported a deficient philosophy—"what is good for the goose is good for the gander." Consequently, women now abandon their husbands and children.

Women in relationships are not safer because of the women's movement. Women still suffer domestic violence. More women today are abandoned to raise children alone. The incidence of sexually transmitted infections is sky rocketing, and in this respect, women bear the brunt with the risk of pelvic infections, infertility, and even cancer. I think it all comes back to contraception and the philosophy behind it.

Many couples whose contraceptives failed accepted the fact they were going to have a child, some even under heroic conditions. But, the philosophy of contraception ultimately comes down to the belief that pregnancy is a failure. The child is a failure. Theresa Wagner has shown how this plays out in the legal arena. I would like to give you my humble opinion about how this is played out in the medical arena.

The first problem is that contraception sees fertility and pregnancy as diseases. But infertility is a disease too. Menopause? Sick. The only time women are not sick is before puberty. Interestingly, pregnancy is the only "disease" that women go out of their way to catch, usually several times. There are those who would say that it is the unwanted pregnancy that is the disease, but then the definition of disease becomes subjective on the part of the patient. Sort of like saying to the doctor, "I don't like that blood pressure. I want my normal blood pressure to be this."

This leads to the second problem. Based on the disease model, oral contraceptives are rooted in the idea that we have the right to ingest powerful chemicals to force our bodies to do what we want. This mentality sees our bodies as things that exist to be used and manipulated to serve our own ends. It's only our minds that are important. If our bodies are things, then the bodies of those around us are things for us to use, especially if that use is mutual. And if that body has less thinking capacity than ours, like the fetus, and if it also happens to interfere with our desires and our ability to control, then we have the right to get rid of it. Parents know who is truly in control when that baby comes—and it isn't us!

We now have a generation of children whose lives were conditional before they were born. Of course many parents would never have an abortion, but these children, were afforded no protection from society if we, their mothers, decided otherwise. That is the insidious nature of choice. And what will their attitude toward us be when we become old or sick and are weak, vulnerable, interfering with their pleasure?

If we use our bodies as things, how can we expect others not to use us as things as well? In fact, that is why there is a debate among feminists as to whether or not prostitution should be legal and acceptable, as long as the woman is not coerced into it. In other words, using our bodies for cash is okay as long as we agree to it.

If we do not respect ourselves, how can we demand that respect from others? And how can we accept ourselves if something so basic to ourselves, our female fertility, is considered disordered.

In the medical community today we have doctors who no longer know how a woman's body functions normally. On a national morning talk show, a female infertility specialist told the audience that all a woman needs to do in order to achieve pregnancy is to have intercourse on the 10-14th day of her cycle. That is good advice for a woman with 28-day cycles. But a woman who has a 25-day cycle and ovulates on day 11 is going to have problems, especially since her most fertile day is day 9. In addition, a woman with a 35-day cycle will never get pregnant following that advice. I have patients who have had multiple cultures performed by gynecologists because of a recurrent "infection" that occurs every month, ending about 2 weeks before her next menses.

Menses itself has become inconvenient, something to be suppressed. We condemn athletes for taking body altering steroids, but for women, that is not only normal, it is expected. Consider also the latest cry of dismay over the fact that a woman's fertility decreases with age. That simple, basic fact has been forgotten. It says volumes. But the response is for technology to improve to the point where woman can just freeze their eggs until they want to use them.

The medical profession, at least at the organizational level, now reflects secular society. Many of my colleagues have swallowed the idea that women's health, by definition, involves the "right" of abortion and contraception. In New York City, abortion is part of the residency program. That is the norm. A resident who chooses not to participate in abortion, must justify his or her decision.

In our country, there is almost a reflexive mocking of Natural Family Planning. Perhaps it is, in part, because we are enamored of all the bells and whistles of modern medicine. Medicine comes out of a disease-based model with disease prevention only recently grafted on. There was a time when a doctor could do only two things in regard to disease—cut it out or hold the patient's hand and let nature take its course. Often we medical personnel watch the monitor instead of the patient, waiting for it to tell us what to do. Even in labor and delivery, we watch the monitor rather that touch the patient's belly.

Obstetrics/gynecology, where many women receive their care, is a surgically-based specialty. Surgeons do their definitive work when patients are under anesthesia. This makes doctors, as a profession, more comfortable with prescribing pills than changing behavior.

Today we expect medicine to give us the ability to determine the condition of our children's conception—despite our advanced age, to select the proper genes to save a sibling. Those that don't match or have the same genetic disorder as the sibling in need are destroyed. The parents justified this as their right, their choice.

Some say that the "excess" embryos from in vitro fertilization should be used to relieve the suffering of others. Some say that about "therapeutic" cloning. Why not let it grow to fetal stage and take its organs? We can do it with cows. A cloned cow was placed into the uterus of another cow. When it was at the fetal stage it was removed and its organs implanted back into the cow from which the clone came, where the organs continued to grow and function. This won't be done with humans they say. Why not? If a couple can choose the child who is genetically the best to save an ill child, why not let them develop a fetus for its organs—after all, it is not a person and therefore has no protection under the law.

Please know that there are many in gynecology who do not espouse this view. And I fault my specialty—family practice—which emphasizes preventive medicine, an outgrowth of the hand holding family doctor. We claim to emphasize the need for preventative health and health preservation—except when it comes to fertility. We recognize that the importance of the person-in-community, especially the family—except when it comes to a woman's decision to have an abortion or a child's right to contraception.

Trying to change patient behavior takes time and its results are less than immediate. It requires that we work with our patients. The ultimate example of how physicians have joined with those who promote contraception is their unwillingness to give women all the information they need to make fully informed decisions regarding their health care. Because women might choose not to take the pill if they were made aware of its mechanism of action, that information is withheld. And not only withheld, but the definition of conception has been changed as well so that doctors can hide behind it. "No, no, dear, that information might upset you." "Let me, your wise doctor make the decision for you." How paternalistic!

So with society's blessing, we take the easy way out. We promote virtue in a pill. Forget diet and exercise—"Lose weight while you sleep." Studies show that teenagers are much less likely to have sexual intercourse if their parents are engaged in their lives and are definite in their expectations (DiClemente 2001). But don't expect to see a Planned Parenthood ad urging parents to talk to their teenagers about abstinence. No, the prevailing wisdom is to assume that teenagers lie about their sexual activity, and girls just need to be put on something so they don't get pregnant—forgetting the other costs, including STDs and the risk of exploitation. Children we do not allow to sign contracts or drive cars are given license to consent to sex.

I testified before the Wisconsin legislature in favor of a bill to allow medical personnel, on the basis of conscience, to decline to prescribe contraception. In response, a female Committee member insisted that if that passed doctors should have to post a sign at the receptionist's desk stating that contraceptives are not provided. NFP providers were to be labeled for not providing complete "reproductive care."

Response to Wagner

Natural Family Planning, on the other hand, says the ebbs and flows of a woman's fertility are normal. Something to be worked with, not suppressed. NFP also recognizes that the mind and body are connected. As a family practitioner, this is the philosophy I trained under. Disease doesn't happen in isolation. Health and illness affects not only the patient, but his or her relationships as well and vice versa. Thus, a family physician must take into consideration how a disease, especially a chronic illness, affects the whole patient: mind, body, and soul. It is also important to be educated to maintain one's health. To that, one needs to know how to take care of their body, to learn how it works. Preventing disease and promoting healthy living of the mind, body, and soul is what is important. NFP makes women partners with their physicians by learning to monitor their own health.

We cooperate with our bodies. We care for our bodies. We respect our bodies. We let no one or nothing else control our bodies, not men, not the government, not drugs. Thus, it boils down to the fundamental difference in how we view the human body, in particular, the woman's body.

The Catholic Church remains consistent in promoting the need to protect the unitive and procreative nature of sexual intercourse. Sadly, within the Church, people in midlevel management responsible for the day-to-day functioning of the Church, do not support the Church's teaching on human sexuality. Those who support the Church's teaching often remain silent. When I was pregnant with my fourth child, my associate pastor, a man I had labeled as "liberal," shocked me when he told me that he supported me, that there were not many couples nowadays who were "courageous" enough to have a large family.

Priests, want to help us to grow closer to God. They also want to be liked. (Don't we all?) They have been told that no one's mind is changed by a homily, so why even try. My reply is that we should plant the seed, water it, help it to bring another's work to fruition. But just bringing up the topics of contraception and abortion can elicit strong feelings from those who do not want to deal with them because that may require them to re-examine their lives. Priests do not like "getting yelled at" anymore than any of us do. How must a priest feel when in the middle of a homily, several people stand up and walk out? It is easier to stick to opposing the death penalty then it is to preach on the immorality of birth control.

We are a generation of Catholics who are doctrinally illiterate. Before we can even begin the battle, we must be trained. We must be taught the why of our beliefs. We must be energized from within and above. As G. K. Chesterton (1993) said in his introduction to *The Everlasting Man*

> . . . children have very little difficulty about the dogmas of the Church. But the Church, being a highly practical thing for working and fighting, is necessarily a thing for men (and women) and not merely for children. There must be in it for working purposes a great deal of tradition, of familiarity, and even of routine. But when its fundamentals are doubted, as at present, we must try to recover the candor and wonder of the child; the unspoilt realism and objectivity of innocence. Or if we cannot do that, we must try at least to shake off the cloud of mere custom and see the thing as new, if only by seeing it as unnatural. Things that may well be familiar so long as familiarity breeds affection, had much better become unfamiliar when familiarity brings contempt...Indeed, contempt must be an illusion. We must invoke the most wild and soaring of imagination; the imagination that can see what is there. (p14)

We need the strong and formal support of our Church to help us evangelize. We must never fear to seek the truth. We need research. And we must ask the questions that need to be asked, to look back at the literature if necessary. Remember the case of the missing criminals? The study purported to show that a drop in the crime rate was due to abortion (Donohue and Levitt 2001). That study showed no association with violent adult behavior, only juvenile delinquency. When the researchers controlled for the environment, i.e., when the children grew up in a stable—two parent home, there was no association at all (Forsman and Thuwe 1966).

We are countercultural and we should take pride in that. As a woman, I am afraid, very afraid, of the utilitarian philosophy which devalues human life and which scientists as well as philosophers like Peter Singer, promote. Hopefully we have been moving away from that philosophy.

We must be patient. We must be wise. Margaret Sanger, in her promotion of free love, eugenics, and planned parenthood accepted many small victories before reaching her goal because she never lost sight of the "big picture." We must do likewise. Change may not come in our lifetime. But we are in God's time. And as the prayer goes, we just have to get out of the way to let Him do what He wants to do with us.

Cynthia Jones-Nosacek, M.D.
Famil Practice and Obstetrics
Columbia-St, Mary's Hospital
Milwaukee, Wisconsin

References

Chesterton, C.K. 1993. *The Everlasting Man*. San Francisco: Ignatius Press, p. 14.

DiClemente, R.J., et al. 2001. "Parent-adolescent communication and sexual risk behaviors among African American adolescent females." *Journal of Pediatrics* 139: 407-412.

Donohue, J. J. & Levitt, S.D., 2001. "The Impact of Legalized Abortion on Crime." *The Quarterly Journal of Economics* 66(2):379-420.

Forsman, H., & Thuwe, I., 1966. "120 Children Born after Application for Therapeutic Abortion Refused." *Acta Psychiatry Scandinavia* 42:71-88.

The Future of Obstetrics and Gynecology:
The right to be trained and practice according to conscience
A Summary Report of an International Conference

Hanna Klaus, M.D.
Executive Director
NFP Center, Washington, DC

MaterCare International and the World Federation of Catholic Medical Associations (FIAMC) convened a conference in Rome in June 2001. I was honored to be one of the presenters and will present a summary of the discussion.

Those who spoke about the right to be trained in Obstetrics and Gynecology according to one's conscience included medical students and residents as well as practicing and retired physicians. They came from the United States, Western and Eastern Europe, Asia, Africa and Australia. All were Roman Catholic and all shared the definition of conscience given in the *Catechism of the Catholic Church*. Despite the multinational profile of the participants, each wished to practice medicine in conformity with such principles as stated for instance in the *Ethical and Religious Directives* of the United States Conference of Catholic Bishops.

Until the paradigm shift in medical ethics, brought about by the acceptance of contraception and, later, abortion, Roman Catholics and those who shared their views on the inviolability of human life were not considered counter-cultural. However, in the last half century, those who refused to condone, let alone participate in abortion were quickly marginalized if they sought admission not only to postgraduate training programs in obstetrics and gynecology, but even entry to medical school. Soon, not-so-subtle discrimination on the part of medical schools extended to those who refused to participate in surgical sterilization or to prescribe contraception.

During the conference, four themes were identified as underlying reasons for the opposition to practice medicine according to conscience: 1) civil law does not protect the right to life of the unborn child; 2) ignorance and misperception about the methods of Natural Family Planning; 3) limits of the health care delivery system; and 4) an inadequate philosophical education for both students and faculty. Remedies were also discussed.

An outline follows per each theme summarizing the central points.

1. Civil law does not protect the right to life of the unborn child

When civil law does not protect the life of the unborn child the following consequences occur:

A. Abortion on demand

B. Manipulation and cannibalization of the human embryo and fetus

C. Coercion of women to abort by

— Boyfriends who do not want to assume the responsibilities of paternity

— Families who for reasons of poverty, limited space or convenience actively object to the ongoing pregnancy and who refuse to assist the pregnant woman in raising her child

— Governments by subtle or overt pressure

— Abortion clinic personnel who are often inadequately trained in counseling and act more like procurers for the clinic's services than professional counselors. (They frequently downplay the gravity of the procedure, fail to offer alternatives honestly, and deny post-abortion grief.)

— Professional marginalization of physicians and nurses who attempt to counter points A, B and C above. (In practice, conscience clauses do not protect physicians, let alone nursing staff who object to abortion, and/or the manipulation of women when they are "counseled" to abort, often in the absence of honest consideration of alternatives.)

2. Ignorance and misperception about the methods of Natural Family Planning

Due to the widespread misperception about the existence, effectiveness and utility of modern methods of Natural Family Planning, the following consequences occur:

A. A patient's choice is limited by only providing contraceptives

B. Most often the effectiveness of contraceptives is exaggerated while neither their side effects nor even their mode of action are fully explained. If a physician is bold enough to offer NFP, he or she is often ridiculed on the grounds that either the methods are not effective, or that the client is incapable of applying them properly.

C. If an NFP-only physician belongs to a "mixed" practice group where other members offer only contraceptives, either the NFP only physician's orders have been changed by colleagues, or patients are steered away from this physician by staff.

3. Limits of the health care delivery system

Various medical practices as well as the structure of patient care itself contribute to creating obstacles to NFP education and instruction. For example,

A. Time constraints of the health care delivery system are well known. This limitation makes it impossible to sufficiently counsel a woman about her medical options—whether they concern family planning or a crisis pregnancy.

B. Rotations for physicians in training affect patient continuity of care. For example, if a doctor begins to teach NFP to a client in the first visit, he or she may not see the client on the next visit. Due to rotations, the next doctor may not know, or care about NFP and the patient is left without adequate training.

C. Mixing surgeries. As far too many Cesarean sections are followed by tubal ligations, the resident who objects to participation may not get an adequate surgical experience. Alternatively, he or she may be allowed to do the section but has to step aside and let another doctor perform the ligation. Not a comfortable situation at best, and always leaves the doctor wondering if his or her preoperative counseling was adequate.

4. Inadequate philosophical/ethical education for both students and faculty

An inadequate philosophical/ethical education in basic principles which should guide professional conduct as well as protect both patient and doctor, is the foundation of the opposition for practicing medicine according to one's conscience. This inadequacy can be grouped as follows:

A. Lack of information regarding ethical and religious directives for hospitals or, worse, efforts to circumvent them by persons in authority. Examples abound in cases of mergers between religious hospitals and secular hospitals. The example of the woman who delivers in the Catholic hospital and then is taken to the non-Catholic "surgicenter" on the same premises for a tubal ligation is well known.

B. The obligation to practice at the level of "reasonable skill and care." This would appear to jeopardize the practicing Catholic who refuses to prescribe contraception. If the playing field were level, which it is not, the obverse would be true: the physician who is ignorant of the efficacy and utility of modern natural methods of family planning would be judged below the threshold of competency.

C. Social and marketing pressure to try to be helpful to patients in accordance with the patient's value system, without averting to the fact that the physician must remain faithful to his or her own value system antecedently.

(1) The doctor-patient relationship is a fiduciary one, even though current terminology tends to mask it by referring to physicians as providers of health care, and patients as consumers.

(2) A patient is, by definition, ill, hence vulnerable and that demands first, recognition of the patient's vulnerability and second, a commitment to serve only the patient's best interests. When there are conflicts, these must be recognized and resolved, without becoming either defensive or confrontational.

(3) It must be observed that fertility is not a disease, hence requires no medical treatment. However, the market forces which attempt to pressure women into ingesting potentially harmful drugs to alter their normal physiological state need to be unmasked and potential users must know the risks they may incur.

5. Projected remedies

A. More residency training programs that allow for practical freedom of conscience without jeopardizing training opportunities. (A great deal depends on the program director, and much more needs to be done.)

B. More physicians have been exposed to NFP delivery systems, broadening the knowledge base considerably.

C. Recognition that fertility is not a disease and that natural regulation of fertility can be learned from a trained instructor who does not need to be a physician or a nurse.

The concept of NFP can be introduced even in the limited time frame of an HMO appointment and referral made for instruction with a certified NFP teacher.

D. Implement standards for NFP teachers. For example, the Diocesan Development Program for NFP, United States Conference of Catholic Bishops, has developed standards for NFP instruction and programs which are professionally acceptable.

E. Fit the needs of the current generation. For example, the NFP Institute of Marquette University in the United States has combined the natural signs of fertility with technical indicators. This is appealing to the younger generation that places value on technology.

F. Proactive chastity education for adolescents which includes fertility awareness.

G. More public enunciation of the value of a conscientious vs. a pragmatic ethical basis for practice.

Response to Dr. Klaus

Dr. Klaus covered a lot of ground in her excellent talk on The Future of Obstetrics & Gynecology –The Right to be Trained and Practice According to Conscience. I have a few comments and observations on the subject.

I, too, am very troubled by the culture and morality that currently prevail in our profession of obstetrics and gynecology. Right now, the point of view is that a patient's autonomy in fertility choices is the only absolute. Contraception, sterilization, artificial insemination, in vitro fertilization, and morning after pills are all taken for granted as good medicine. Abortion is viewed as sometimes unpleasant but necessary and certainly every woman's right. Prenatal diagnosis of Down syndrome is now a huge industry in which the most highly trained OB doctors known as Maternal Fetal Medicine Specialists, spend their days doing ultrasounds and amniocentises. "Standard of Care," according to the American College of Obstetrics and Gynecology is to offer screening for Down syndrome to every patient. Refusal to do so on the part of an OB or midwife risks a lawsuit for "wrongful life" if a child with Down's goes undetected and is born.

The whole specialty of Maternal-Fetal Medicine or Perinatology, as it is often called, is so steeped in eugenics that several years ago, an opinion piece in a major journal argued that a pro-life physician could not maintain his or her integrity in this specialty and should therefore get out (Blustein and Fleishman 1995).

In spite of all these bad things, I think there are some reasons for hope.

1. First of all, in the United States, apparently more so than in Europe and other parts of the world, freedom of conscience even for a health care provider is still held in high esteem. Recently, for example, a U.S. district court in Riverside, California ruled in favor of a nurse who refused to prescribe or dispense morning after pills. She had been fired because of her refusal and the court awarded her back pay and emotional damages of $47,000.

My impression is that most OB residents in the U.S. are not marginalized for refusing to do abortions as apparently they are in Europe. Those who won't prescribe contraception, I think, face greater discrimination.

Response to Klaus   77

However, some certainly have succeeded in getting through OB/GYN residencies. Two of those physicians practice in Milwaukee and both finished their residencies with honors in the last decade.

2. I am also hopeful about the future because in recent years I have seen more interest among medical students in the area of medical ethics. Students tend to challenge the status quo, and the contraceptive mentality is certainly the status quo. Recently, a group of medical students refused to give Depo-Provera contraceptive injections at a local Catholic hospital, expressing surprise that it was allowed at a Catholic hospital. Other students have raised questions about the ethics of prenatal diagnosis of Down syndrome.

3. A third reason for hope as far as freedom of conscience goes, is that training programs in the fields of OB/GYN and Family Practice are having trouble filling their spots nation wide the last few years. Residency directors are less likely to discriminate if it means there will be a vacancy in their program.

4. I also think there is growing organized support for pro-life medical students and residents from groups such as Physicians Alliance. The American Association of Prolife OB/GYNs and One More Soul both publish directories of Pro-Life and NFP-only physicians allowing residents to connect with like-minded mentors. And I think the number of NFP only physicians is growing, albeit slowly. Here in Milwaukee's OB/GYN residency there are three NFP-only OB/GYNs on the faculty teaching medical students and residents.

Although there are hurdles in the road for those who want to be trained and practice according to their conscience, there is reason to be optimistic.

One final thought: although discrimination against those who are faithful to Catholic teaching on reproductive issues is a problem, the greater problem is the Church's failure to properly form consciences in this area. Here's what I mean. About 25% of OB residents are nominally Catholic. 3-4% of Catholics use NFP. Therefore, only about 1% of OB residents can be expected to be committed to the Church's teaching on contraception and sterilization. That means that in an OB Residency like Milwaukee's, which has 6 residents per year, we can expect an NFP only OB/GYN once every 17 years. The Church has to do a better job of catechizing its members and bringing its truths to a mixed up culture.

James Linn, M.D.
Obstetrics/Gynecology
Columbia-St. Mary's Hospital, Milwaukee

Reference

Blustein, J., and Fleishman, A.R. 1995. "The Pro-Life Maternal-Fetal Medicine Physician: A Problem of Integrity." *Hastings Center Report* 5: 22-26.

Day-Specific Probabilities of Conception in the Menstrual Cycle

Joseph B. Stanford, M.D., M.S.P.H.
Department of Family and Preventive Medicine,
University of Utah
and

David B. Dunson, Ph.D.
Biostatistics Branch, National Institute of
Environmental Health Sciences

The concept of day-specific probabilities of conception is receiving increased attention in clinical, epidemiologic, demographic and statistical research. It offers important insights into our fundamental biologic understanding of human fertility and gives us a precise research tool to examine the effects of environment, drugs, or chemicals on human fertility. It has great potential to improve the diagnosis and treatment of infertility. Natural family planning (NFP) has a lot to offer in methods, data, and interpretation with regard to day-specific probabilities of conception. In the process, we can also gain a better understanding of the effectiveness of NFP to avoid and to achieve pregnancy.

Definitions of Terms of Reproductive Capacity
In order to discuss the concept of day-specific probabilities of conception, we first need to set forth its definition and the definitions of several related measures of human reproductive capacity. The relationship between these various measures are illustrated in Figure 1.

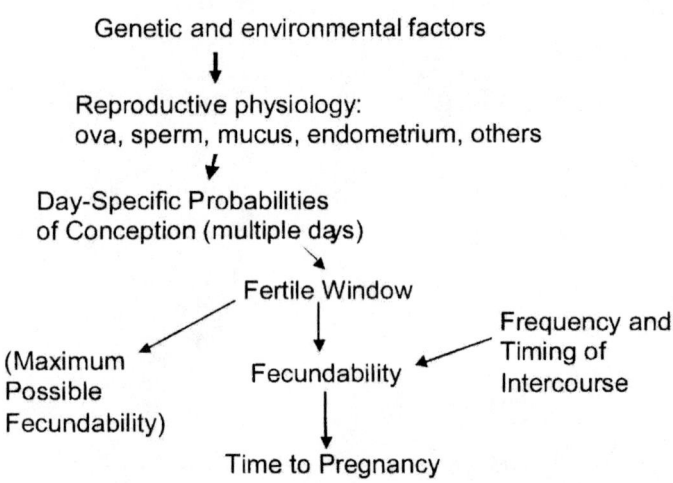

Figure 1. Relationship of various measures of reproductive capacity, physiology, genetic, environmental factors, and the frequency and timing of intercourse.

Pregnancy can be defined as beginning at fertilization (the uniting of the sperm and the egg) or at implantation (when the embryo attaches to the uterine lining). While there is no question that the process of development of a new human individual begins at conception (fertilization), there are no reliable measures available to detect this event. Some researchers have flushed early embryos out of the fallopian tubes (Alvarez, Guiloff et al. 1988) but this procedure obviously has severe ethical objections. For research purposes, a reliable means of identifying the occurrence of pregnancy is needed. Currently, the most reliable way to detect early pregnancy is the measurement of human chorionic gonadotropin (hCG), the pregnancy hormone produced by the embryo and trophoblast. This can detect pregnancy around the time of implantation (Wilcox, Weinberg et al. 1985). Studies that have been conducted using hCG suggest that 22% of pregnancies end before the woman recognizes that she is pregnant (Wilcox and Weinberg et al. 1988).

More commonly in research and in clinical practice, pregnancy is defined simply by women recognizing signs of pregnancy in their bodies, including an absence of expected menstruation. This is called "clinically evident pregnancy." In NFP, we often define pregnancy based on criteria applied to NFP charts: e.g., 19 to 21 days of postovulatory phase following the mucus peak day or of a basal body temperature hyperthermic phase. It seems likely that women using NFP will recognize some early pregnancies that end in miscarriage (spontaneous abortion) that women not using NFP would not recognize, but this has not been definitively studied. Clinically evident pregnancies may also be confirmed by urine testing for hCG, which is widely available over-the-counter. For the rest of this paper, we will focus on clinically evident pregnancy as our definition of pregnancy. For the purposes of this paper, "conception" is considered to have occurred if there is subsequent recognition of a clinically recognized pregnancy.

A ***day-specific probability of conception*** can be defined as the probability of conception (or clinically recognized pregnancy) occurring if sexual intercourse were to occur only on a specific day of the menstrual cycle. This day is referenced according to the estimated day of ovulation, which is designated as day 0. For example, the day occurring 3 days before the day of ovulation is designated day −3, and the day occurring 4 days after the day of ovulation is designated day +4.

Day-specific probabilities of conception are dependent on the viability (or "life span") of the ovum and the sperm. These in turn are related to reproductive hormones, receptors, and physiologic processes. As those familiar with NFP know, cervical mucus plays an essential role in the viability span of the sperm. Ultimately, all of these processes are influenced by genetic factors (both female and male) and environmental factors. (See Figure 1.)

The ***fertile window*** is the consecutive period of time in the menstrual cycle during which sexual intercourse results in a significant probability of pregnancy. This includes all days in which there is a significant day-specific probability of conception. For practical reasons, this is measured in days, rather than hours. The fertile window has been found to be about 6 days long in most studies. (This will vary a little depending on the cutoff one uses for a significant probability of conception- e.g., a cutoff of 0.1% for day-specific probabilities of conception will give wider window than a cutoff of 5% for day-specific probabilities of conception.) Like day-specific probabilities of conception, the reference point for the fertile window is the estimated day of ovulation.

Maximum possible fecundability is the highest possible probability of conception if intercourse were to occur on every day during the fertile window. In other words, if there is intercourse on every possibly fertile day, maximum possible fecundability is the highest possible probability that pregnancy could occur. Maximum possible fecundability reflects the underlying fertile potential of the couple. It is obviously dependent on the fertile window. It will vary between populations. For example, as will be discussed later in this paper, an older population will have decreased maximum possible fecundability. Importantly, it also varies considerably within the same population. In other words, some couples really are more fertile than others.

Fecundability is the actual probability of conception for a single menstrual cycle. The difference between fecundability and maximum possible fecundability is the couple's sexual behavior. In other words, when the couple has intercourse during the fertile window will determine how close the fecundability of that cycle gets to maximum possible fecundability.

Time to pregnancy is a measure of reproductive capacity that is often used in research studies. It is usually defined as the number of menstrual cycles of noncontracepted intercourse it takes for a couple to get pregnant. Time to pregnancy is a direct function of fecundability. As such, it is also dependent on when the couple has intercourse during the fertile window.

Reproductive Physiology

As Figure 1 illustrates, there are a number of physiologic processes in both the female and the male that determine the day-specific probabilities of conception, and therefore the fertile window. First, the length of time that an ovum can be fertilized has been shown by many different studies to be quite limited after ovulation occurs, certainly less than a day, and probably on the order of a few hours (Dunson, Weinberg et al. 2001; Yuzpe, Albert et al 2000; Harrison 1988). The major determinant of the length of the fertile window, then, is how long a sperm remains viable. As those familiar with NFP know well, how long a sperm remains viable depends in turn on the presence or absence of Type E (estrogenic) mucus produced by the uterine cervix (Hilgers and Prebil 1979; Billings, Billings et al. 1989; Odeblad 1997).

As noted earlier, day-specific probabilities of conception are indexed to the key event of ovulation. There are a number of biological markers that can be used to estimate the day of ovulation (Stanford, White et al. 2002). Among these are the peak day of mucus discharge, the thermal shift in basal body temperature, and the assessment of the ratio of estrogen metabolites to progesterone metabolites in the urine. Other measures could potentially be used, but in this paper we will restrict our attention to those just listed, because they have been actually used in studies of day-specific probabilities of conception. Each of the methods listed has certain advantages and disadvantages, and each has some error in identifying the day of ovulation, i.e., it may be one or more days different from the actual day of ovulation (Dunson and Weinberg 2000).

Research Questions about the Fertile Window

The rest of this paper will develop the concept of day-specific probabilities of conception, with the goal of answering the following questions about the fertile window:

1) How many days during a menstrual cycle can intercourse result in pregnancy?
2) Which of these days has the highest probability of pregnancy?
3) Does the fertile window vary by age?
4) How much variation is there in the fertile window between couples?
5) Does the fertile window vary by drug exposure?
6) How can women identify their own fertile window prospectively?
7) How does the fertile window change in sub-fertile couples?

In order to answer these questions, we need data and statistical methods to analyze those data in terms of day-specific probabilities of conception. The data that are needed are a marker of ovulation (as discussed above), accurate daily records of intercourse (and contraceptive use, if any), and good follow up to ascertain outcome (conception, here defined as clinically evident pregnancy). There are a few data sets that meet these requirements and have been used to calculate day-specific probabilities. These are outlined in Table 1. It is notable that three of the four data sets come from groups of NFP users. Specifically, the Barrett-Marshall data set comes from 241 users of the Basal Body Temperature Method in England (Barrett and Marshall 1969), the European fecundability data set comes from 782 users of the Sympto-Thermal Method in 7 different European centers in 6 different European countries (Colombo and Masarotto 2000), and the Creighton Model Fertility*Care*™ System data set comes from 6 different Creighton Model Centers in 4 different states of the United States (Stanford and Smith 2000). The sole exception, the North Carolina data set, was based on women or couples who wanted to get pregnant, and who kept daily records of intercourse and collected daily urine samples, from which the timing of ovulation was determined retrospectively, without the prior knowledge of the women (Wilcox, Weinberg et al. 1995). It is also worth noting that only one of the data sets has included couples with known infertility, namely the Creighton Model Fertility*Care*™ System data set. The other three data sets were designed to include only couples that were of apparently normal fertility.

Not included in table 1 are a data set that was based on artificial insemination rather than natural intercourse (Schwartz and Mayaux 1982), and another data set that had some significant methodologic problems with regard to the type of analyses is discussed here (Vollman 1977). It should be noted that other data sets are in existence or being developed that may in the future be used to estimate day-specific probabilities of conception. These include another data set from China that is very similar to the North Carolina data set, but larger; a data set based on users of the Sympto-Thermal Method in Germany (Gnoth, Frank-Herrmann et al. 1995); a data set based on 4 Italian centers for the Billings Ovulation Method; and data from users of the ClearPlan® Easy Fertility Monitor or Persona® in England. Data are also being assembled from users of the Ovarian Monitor in Australia and New Zealand. Further, a number of studies have been done in the past that could be analyzed in this way, but for one reason or another, never have been (Hakim, Gray et al. 1994; Eskenazi, Gold et al. 1995; Waller, Reim et al. 1996).

Day-Specific Probabilities of Conception in the Menstrual Cycle

Table 1. Data Sets that Have Been Used to Assess Day-Specific Probabilities

Principal Investigators (Year)	Women/Couples Studied	Ovulation Marker	Number of Women/ Couples	Number of Cycles	Number of Clinical Pregnancies
Barrett, Marshall (1969)	BBT method users in England (all initially avoiding pregnancy)	BBT shift	241	1898	103
Wilcox, Baird, Weinberg (1995)	Women in North Carolina who wanted to get pregnant	Urine estrogen/ progesterone ratio	221	696	144
Colombo, Masarotto, et al (2000)	Sympto-thermal method users in Europe (almost all initially avoiding pregnancy)	BBT shift and mucus peak day	782	5390	434
Stanford, Smith, Dunson (2000)	Creighton Model System users in the U.S.A. including those initially avoiding and achieving pregnancy	Mucus peak day	426	2054	111

Statistical Models

Most cycles that are available from these data sets for analysis have multiple acts of intercourse in the days surrounding the estimated day of ovulation. Therefore, day-specific probabilities of conception cannot be measured directly, but must be estimated by statistical modeling based on a large group of menstrual cycles. Each menstrual cycle analyzed includes intercourse on different days during the cycle. Some cycles result in conception, while others do not. The statistical model analyzes the patterns to extract the "best possible explanation" of the observed probabilities conception relative to when intercourse occurred in each cycle. Several statistical models have been developed for this purpose. Here we review three groups of models: the Schwartz model, several enhancements of the Schwartz model, and the Dunson model (a Bayesian model).

The Schwartz model, first proposed in 1980, is perhaps the most widely used statistical model used to date to estimate day-specific probabilities of conception (Schwartz, MacDonald et al. 1980). It was based on an enhancement of an original model proposed by Barrett and Marshall (Barrett and Marshall 1969). The Schwartz model can be stated mathematically as follows:

Probability (conception | $X_{-5},...,X_0$) = $A\{ 1 - \Pi_k (1-p_k)^{X_k}\}$

Where

A = Probability that the cycle is viable, essentially the same as maximum fecundability

X represents intercourse (0 or 1) on different days in the fertile window

k is an index for the different days of the fertile window

And therefore

Ap_k = Probability of conception if intercourse occurs only on day k

The Schwartz model makes a number of assumptions. The first is that different batches of sperm (from different acts of intercourse) compete independently to fertilize the ovum. In other words, an act of intercourse does not in of itself become more fertile if there are other acts of intercourse before or after (although the multiple acts of intercourse do raise the probability of pregnancy overall in the cycle). This is a reasonable assumption that seems to fit the data that are currently available. The second assumption is that all couples have the same day-specific probabilities of conception in a menstrual cycle. This assumption is more problematic and is probably wrong. There is likely to be quite a bit of variability in fertility and potential fertility between different couples within a population. Some of this variation may be explained by factors that can be easily measured (such as age), and some of it may not be easily explained. There may also be day-specific information (e.g., quality of cervical mucus discharge on that day) other than timing relative to ovulation that the Schwartz model cannot account for. The model also assumes that the fertile window is the same number of days for each couple. Finally, a significant problem with the Schwartz model is that it can be considered statistically imprecise. That is, there are so many parameters in the model to estimate that it is difficult to apply the model without a large set of cycles, and even then, the confidence intervals for the day-specific probabilities tend to be wide.

The Schwartz model has been modified to address some of these limitations and to make other enhancements. For example, it has been modified to allow covariate effects on A (Weinberg, Gladen et al. 1994), covariate effects on p_k (Zhou and Weinberg 1996), variability among couples in A (Zhou, Weinberg et al. 1996), account for missing data regarding intercourse (Dunson and Weinberg 2000a), and adjust for measurement error in identifying the true day of ovulation (Dunson and Weinberg 2000b) (Dunson, Weinberg et al. 2001a), as well as other enhancements (Dunson, Weinberg et al. 2001b; Royston and Ferreira 1999).

To overcome deficiencies of the Schwartz model more systematically, Dunson developed a Bayesian model for day-specific probabilities of conception (Dunson 2001). This model can be stated mathematically as follows:

Probability (conception in cycle j from couple i | X) =
$A_{ij}[\ X_{ijM} + (1-X_{ijM})\{\ 1 - \Pi(1-p_{ijl})^{X_{ij,l+M}}\ \}]$
Where
A = Probability that the cycle is viable
X represents intercourse (0 or 1) for couple i, cycle j, day l+M
M represents the most fertile day
l is a marker for the different days of the fertile window relative to the most fertile day
A_{ij} = probability of pregnancy if intercourse occurs on the most fertile day.

The Dunson model makes the biologically reasonable assumptions that there is a single day in the menstrual cycle on which the probability of conception is highest (day M), that if intercourse occurs on this day the maximum probability of conception is reached for that cycle, and that the probability of conception increases over the days immediately before and decreases over the days immediately after this "maximum probability" day. This presumption is consistent with all analyses to date that have used the Schwartz model. The model allows different couples to have different fertility levels (i.e., different maximum fecundability), and also different numbers of days in the fertile window. The model can incorporate couple-level variables affecting fertility (e.g., age), and can also incorporate day-specific variables affecting fertility (e.g., quality of mucus discharge).

In the remainder of this paper, we will discuss the use of the Schwartz and Dunson models to answer the specific research questions enumerated earlier.

How many days during a menstrual cycle can intercourse result in pregnancy, and which of these days has the highest probability of pregnancy?

Wilcox et al, using a Schwartz model and the North Carolina data (Table 1), reported that there was a six-day fertile window (the five days up to ovulation and the estimated day of ovulation itself) during which intercourse could result in pregnancy (Wilcox, Weinberg et al. 1995). This is probably the best known and most widely quoted application of modeling day-specific probabilities of conception. The highest probability of conception was on the estimated day of ovulation itself, about 0.33. However, it is important to note that this analysis included pregnancies that were only detected by hCG and not ever detected clinically (i.e., it included pregnancies that resulted in early unrecognized pregnancy loss). In a later analysis based on clinically recognized pregnancies and using a modified Schwartz model, the highest probability of conception (with clinically identified pregnancy) for both the North Carolina and the England data (Table 1) was found to occur 1-2 days prior to ovulation, rather than the day of ovulation itself (see Figure 2) (Dunson, Baird et al. 1999). It is also important to note that the six-day fertile window is not absolute. Analyses of the substantially larger European data set, both with the Schwartz model (Colombo and Masarotto 2000), and with the Dunson model (Dunson, Colombo et al. 2002), have found much smaller but still nonzero probabilities of conception from intercourse more than 5 days before the estimated day of ovulation. In other words, intercourse on day 6 or 7 prior to the estimated day of ovulation may rarely result in pregnancy. How much of this may be due to occasional prolonged sperm survival, and how much may be due to errors in identifying the day of ovulation is not known at this time. Although there is some error in identifying the exact day of ovulation, the available data is fully consistent with the hypothesis that conception never occurs the day after ovulation.

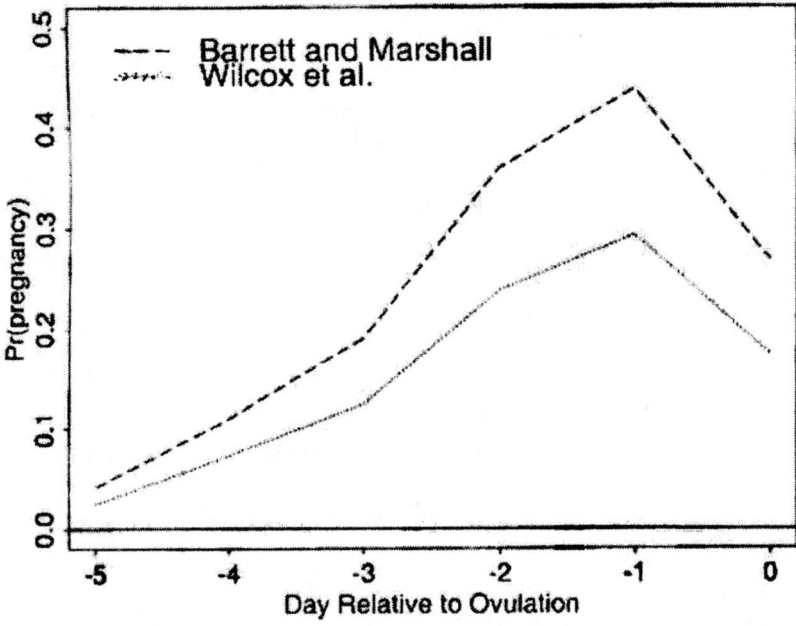

Figure 2. Estimated probablility of achieving a clinicial pregnancy based on a single act of intercourse in each study. The dashed line represents the estimates from the Barrett and Marshall cohort, and the dotted line represent the estimates from the Wilcox *et. al.* cohort.

Does the fertile window vary by age?
While a number of studies in the past have shown that fertility declines with female age, the question remains as to how much of this decline is due to actual decreases in fecundity, and how much is due to decreased frequency of intercourse. To sort this out, a study of day-specific probabilities of pregnancy is needed. Dunson, Columbo, et al recently published an analysis of day-specific probabilities relative to maternal and paternal age. This was based on the European Sympto-thermal data set (Table 1) and used the Dunson statistical model (Dunson, Colombo et al. 2002). Figure 3 shows the results. On average, women aged 19-26 had a maximum probability of getting pregnant of over 50%, 2 days prior to the estimated day of ovulation (in this case, the last day of low basal body temperatures, so this was 3 days prior to

the first day of temperature rise). However, women aged 35-39, on average, had a maximum probability of getting pregnant of less than 30%, again 3 days prior to the first day of temperature rise.

What about the effect of men's age? Because husbands and wives are usually within a few years of each other's age, this is a more difficult question to examine with the available data. However, the same study was also able to examine this question for husbands who were 5 years older than their wives (Dunson, Colombo et al. 2002). The results of this analysis are shown in Figure 4. For younger women, there is little effect of the man being 5 years or more older. However, for women aged 35-39, there is a significant additional drop in the probability of conception if the man is 5 years or more older. It is interesting that even though there was a drop in day-specific probabilities of conception for both men and women, the length of the fertile window in days remained unchanged.

It is important to emphasize that this was not a study of infertility. In fact, infertile couples (where known), were excluded from this European data set. Just because older couples who take longer to get pregnant does not necessarily mean that they ultimately cannot get pregnant, even though it may take longer.

What is the cause of the decline in fertility with age? This is not known completely, but it seems likely that decreased ovarian function and decreased number of available ova in older women as well as decreased viability of sperm in older men (including an increase in genetic abnormalities of sperm) both play a role. This is consistent with these analyses. (See Figures 3–4)

How much variation is there in the fertile window between couples?

Earlier, we noted that there is some variability between couples in their ability to achieve pregnancy, even if none of the couples have a history of infertility. The study previously mentioned also examined this question (Dunson, Colombo et al. 2002). The results are shown in Figure 5. It seems that there is a very large amount of variability in day-specific probabilities of conception and maximum fecundability, even among couples who have no history of infertility. For example, couples in the 95th percentile (in other words, out of 100 couples of apparently normal fertility, the 5% most fertile couples), have a maximum probability of conception of over 85% if they have intercourse on the most fertile day. On the other hand, couples in the 5th percentile (in other words, out of 100 couples of apparently

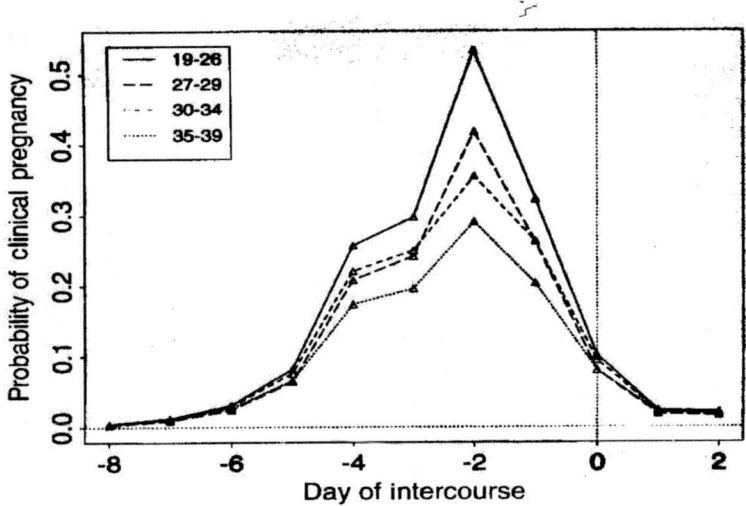

Figure 3. Day-specific probabilities of conception according to age of the woman, based on analysis of the European fecundability database.

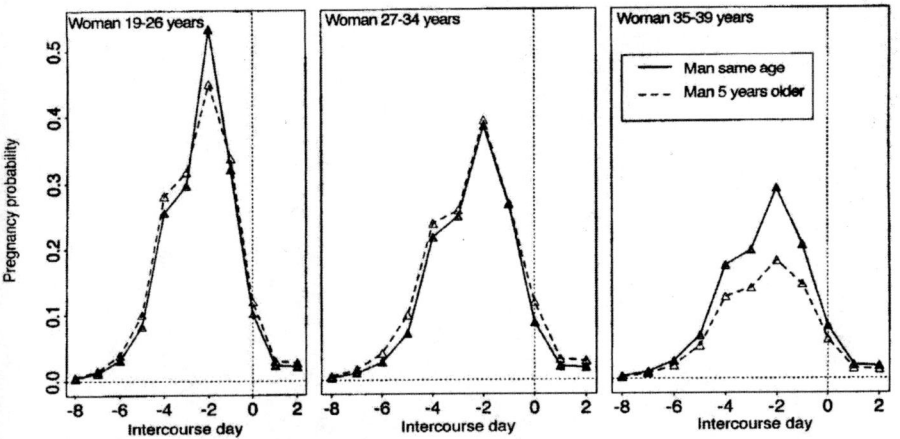

Figure 4. Relationship of day-specific probabilities of conception to the difference between the man's and the woman's age.

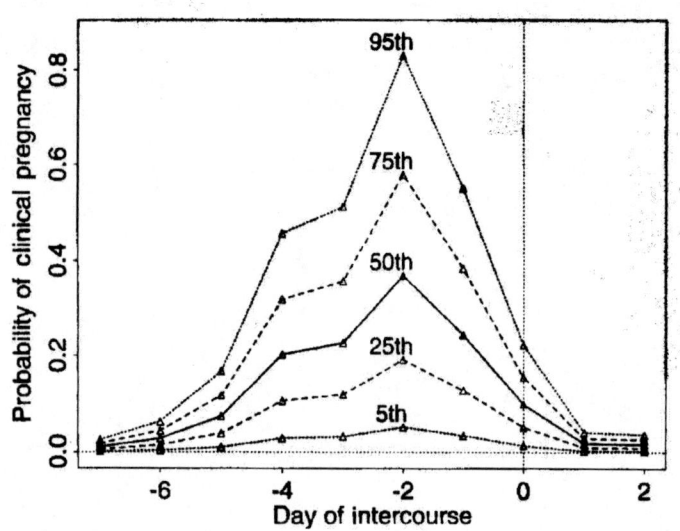

Figure 5. Variability of day-specific probabilities of conception within a normally fertile population.

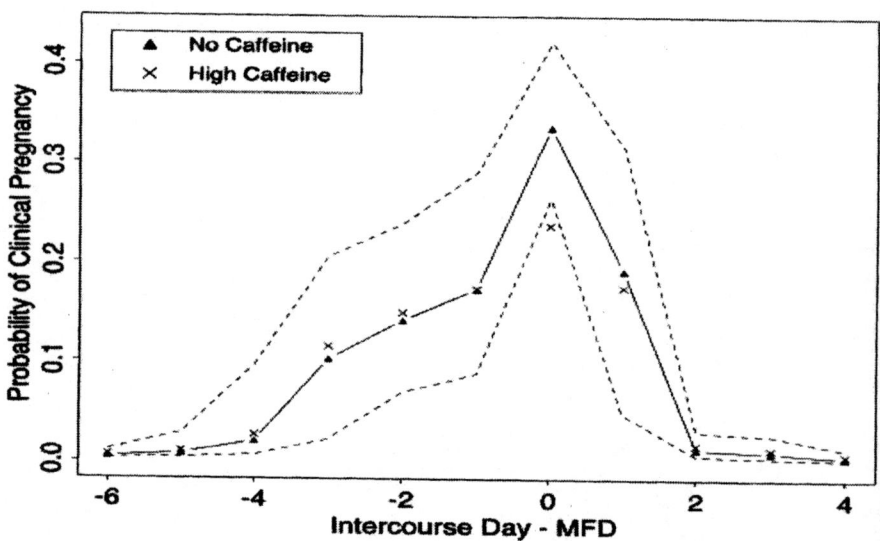

Figure 6. Day-specific probabilities of conception in relation to caffeine intake equivalent of about 2 cups or more coffee per day.

normal fertility, the 5 least fertile couples), have a maximum probability of conception of less than 5% if they have intercourse on the most fertile day of the cycle. Similarly, couples at the 75th percentile have a maximum probability of conception close to 60% and couples at the 25th percentile have a maximum probability of conception a little less than 20%.

Does the fertile window vary by drug exposure?
The Dunson statistical model can be used to examine the effect of drug exposure on both the maximum probability of conception in the menstrual cycle, and the length (in days) of the fertile window. This has been done using the North Carolina dataset for exposure to caffeine, an area that has been somewhat controversial (Dunson 2001). The results are shown in Figure 6. This analysis suggests that women who drink 2 or more cups of coffee per day (or equivalent) have a reduced maximum probability of conception on the most fertile day, but that the fertile window otherwise remains unchanged.

How can women identify their own fertile window prospectively?
Analyses of both the European fecundability dataset (Colombo and Masarotto 2000; Dunson, Sinai et al. 2001) and the Creighton Model data set (Stanford, Smith, et al. 2003) confirm in empirical data what has been biologically supported for many years (Billings, Brown et al. 1972; Odeblad 1997; Hilgers and Prebil, 1979): the appearance and development of the mucus symptoms is a highly accurate way for women to identify the approach of ovulation and the most fertile days of the menstrual cycle. Changes in the vaginal discharge of cervical mucus have a good correlation with ovulation, precede ovulation, identify the rise in estrogen associated with folliculogenesis (the development of the follicle prior to ovulation), give information about sperm survival, correlate with endocervical mucus sampling, are usually simple to observe and interpret, and are easily learned by women (World Health Organization 1981).

How does the fertile window change in sub-fertile couples?
An analysis of the Creighton Model database shows that the length of the fertile period is similar in couples with sub-fertility (or "infertility"),

but that the maximum probability of pregnancy (the maximum possible fecundability) is greatly reduced (Stanford, Smith, et al. 2003). This analysis suggests that sub-fertile couples can also identify the days in which they are most likely to get pregnant by monitoring the cervical mucus symptom, even though their maximum possible fecundability is less than that of couples with normal fertility.

Conclusion

Day-specific probabilities of conception are an exciting new field of science that has the potential to help us learn much more about human reproduction than we have ever known before. Some of what we are learning is not particularly surprising to NFP users, but other things may be. To summarize what we have learned so far:

1) The fertile window is relatively narrow, regardless of what markers of ovulation are used to assess it.

2) Drugs such as caffeine can affect day-specific probabilities of conception in subtle but important ways.

3) Day-specific probabilities of conception are necessary to fully understand effects of drugs or environment on fertility.

4) There seems to be a steady, gradual decline in fertility (maximum possible fecundability) as females and males age.

5) There is a lot of variation in fertility (maximum possible fecundability) between different couples, even those of the same age and socioeconomic status

6) Day-specific probabilities of conception can be identified by clinical observation of vaginal discharge from cervical mucus.

7) Sub-fertile couples have fecund intervals similar to normally fertile couples, although the day-specific probabilities are much less.

Studies from NFP users have led the way in this field of science. Perhaps this is because the concept of day-specific pregnancy probabilities is a natural part of our way of thinking to NFP users and NFP researchers, since we know with reasonable certainty when ovulation occurs during the menstrual cycle. For those less familiar with NFP, the concept of day-specific probabilities of conception may take some getting used to.

Future Research Questions

Questions to be addressed by future research include

1) What causes the large variation in fertility (maximum possible fecundability) between couples, other than age?

2) What information does the quality of mucus discharge give with regard to other fertility factors and outcomes of pregnancy? This is an active area of research at the Pope Paul VI Institute for the Study of Human Reproduction, where among other things, blood hormone levels and follicular ultrasound are being used to study these questions.

3) How do other drugs and environmental exposures affect day specific probabilities of conception?

4) Do factors that affect fertility affect later outcomes of pregnancy or childhood?

Acknowledgements

Colleagues for Dr. Dunson and Dr. Stanford who were involved in the research summarized in this paper include Allen Wilcox, M.D., Claire Weinberg, Ph.D., Donna Baird, Ph.D., Bernardo Colombo, Ph.D., and Ken Smith, Ph.D. Thomas W. Hilgers, M.D. and James Trussell, Ph.D., were consultants for the Creighton Model Fecundity Study.

Participating European Centers for the European Fecundability Study:
Centro Ambrosiano Metodi Naturali, Milan, Italy
Instituto per l'Educazione alla Sessualita e alla Fertilita, Verona, Italy
Natuerliche Familienplanung, Frauenklinik, University of Duesseldorf, Germany
Fertility U.K., London, United Kingdom
Centro Metodi Naturali di Lugano, Lugano, Switzerland
Centre de Liaison des Equipes de Recherche, Paris, France
Federation Francophone pour le Planning Familial Naturel, Couple-Armor-Fecundite, Brussels, Belgium

Participating Creighton Model Centers for the Creighton Model Fecundity Study:

St. John's Mercy Hospital, Department of Fertility Care Services, St. Louis, MO
St. Joseph's Hospital, Department of Women's Health, St. Louis, MO
St. Mary's Health Center, The Women's Well, St. Louis, MO
Fertility Care Services of Nebraska, Lincoln, NE
Fertility Care Services of Wichita, KS
Seton Medical Center Fertility Care Center, Daly City, CA

Note on Figures

Figure 2 comes from Figure 2 in the following paper:
Dunson D, Baird D, Wilcox A, Weinberg C. "Day-specific probabilities of clinical pregnancy based on two studies with imperfect measures of ovulation." *Human Reproduction* 1999; 14:1835-9. Reprinted with permission.

Figure 3 comes from Figure 1 in the following paper:
Dunson D, Colombo B, Baird D. "Changes with age in the level and duration of fertility in the menstrual cycle." *Human Reproduction* 2002; 17:1399-1403. Reprinted with permission.

Figure 4 comes from Figure 2 in the following paper:
Dunson D, Colombo B, Baird D. "Changes with age in the level and duration of fertility in the menstrual cycle." *Human Reproduction* 2002; 17:1399-1403. Reprinted with permission.

Figure 5 comes from Figure 3 in the following paper:
Dunson D, Colombo B, Baird D. "Changes with age in the level and duration of fertility in the menstrual cycle." *Human Reproduction* 2002; 17:1399-1403. Reprinted with permission.

Figure 6 comes from Figure 2 in the following paper:
Dunson D.B. "Bayesian modeling of the level and duration of fertility in the menstrual cycle." *Biometrics* 2001; 57:1067-1073. Reprinted with permission.

Bibliography

Alvarez, F., Guiloff, E. et al. 1988. "New insights on the mode of action of intrauterine contraceptive devices in women." *Fertility and Sterility* 49 (5): 768-73.

Barrett, J.C., and Marshall, J. 1969. "The risk of conception on different days of the menstrual cycle." *Population Studies* 23 (3): 455-461.

Billings, E.L., Billings, J.J. et al. 1989. *Billings Atlas of the Ovulation Method.* Melbourne: Ovulation Method Research and Reference Centre of Australia.

Billings, E.L., Brown, J.B. et al. 1972. "Symptoms and hormonal changes accompanying ovulation." *Lancet* 1 Feb: 282-284.

Colombo, B. and Masarotto, G. 2000. "Daily fecundability: First results from a new database." *Demographic Research* 3 (5).

Dunson, D., Baird, D. et al. 1999. "Day-specific probabilities of clinical pregnancy based on two studies with imperfect measures of ovulation." *Human Reprodution* 14 (7): 1835-9.

Dunson, D., Colombo, B. et al. 2002. "Changes with age in the level and duration of fertility in the menstrual cycle." *Human Reproduction* 17 (5): 1399-1403.

Dunson, D., Sinai, I. et al. 2001. "The Relationship between cervical secretions and the daily probabilities of pregnancy: effectiveness of the TwoDay Algorithm." *Human Reproduction* 16 (11): 2278-2282.

Dunson, D., Weinberg, C. et al. 2001. "Assessing human fertility using several markers of ovulation." *Statistics and Medicine* 20: 965-968.

———. 2001. "Modeling multiple ovulation, fertilization, and embryo loss in human fertility studies." *Biostatistics* 2: 131-145.

Dunson, D.B. 2001. "Bayesian modeling of the level and duration of fertility in the menstrual cycle." *Biometrics* 57: 1067-1073.

Dunson, D.B. and Weinberg, C.R. 2000. "Accounting for unreported and missing intercourse in human fertility studies." *Statistics and Medicine* 19 (5): 665-79.

———. 2000. "Modeling human fertility in the presence of measurement error." *Biometrics* 56 (1): 288-92.

Eskenazi, B., Gold, E.B. et al. 1995. "Prospective assessment of fecundability of female semiconductor workers." *American Journal of Internal Medicine* 28 (6): 817-31.

Gnoth, C., Frank-Herrmann, P. et al. 1995. "The sexual behavior of natural family planning users and its changes in the course of time." *Advances in Contraception* 11 (1): 17.

Hakim, R.B., Gray, R.H. et al. 1994. "Infertility and early pregnancy loss." *American Journal of Obstetrics and Gynecology* 172 (5): 1510-7.

Harrison K.L., Breen, W.L. et al. 1988. "Fertilization of human oocytes in relation to varying delay before insemination." *Fertility and Sterility* 50: 294-297

Hilgers, T.W. and Prebil, A.M. 1979. "The ovulation method—vulvar observations as an index of fertility/infertility." *Obstetrics and Gynecology* 53 (1) Jan: 12-22.

Odeblad, E. 1997. "Cervical mucus and their functions." *Journal of the Irish Colleges of Physicians and Surgeons* 26 (1): 27-32.

Royston, P. and Ferreira, A. 1999. "A new approach to modeling daily probabilities of conception." *Biometrics* 55 (4): 1005-13.

Schwartz, D., MacDonald, P.D.M. et al. 1980. "Fecundability, coital frequency, and the viability of ova." *Population Studies* 34: 397-400

Schwartz, D. and Mayaux, M.J. 1982. "Female fecundity as a function of age: results of artificial insemination in 2193 nulliparous women with azoospermic husbands. Federation CECOS." *New England Journal of Medicine* 306 (7): 404-6.

Stanford, J. B. and Smith, K.R. 2000. "Characteristics of women associated with continuing instruction in the Creighton Model FertilityCare™ System." *Contraception* 61 (2): 121-129.

Stanford, J.B., White, G.L. et al. 2002. "Timing intercourse to achieve pregnancy: current evidence." *Obstetrics and Gynecology* 100: 1333-41.

Stanford, J.B., Smith, K.R., et al. 2003. "Vulvar mucus observation and the probability of pregnancy." *Obstetrics and Gynecology* 101: 1285-93.

Vollman, R.F. 1977. *The menstrual cycle*. Philadelphia, PA:W.B. Saunders.

Waller, K., Reim, J. et al. 1996. "Bone Mass and Subtle Abnormalities in Ovulatory Function in Healthy Women." *Journal of Clinical Endocrinology and Metabolism* 81 (2): 663-668.

Weinberg, C.R., Gladen, B.C. et al. 1994. "Models relating the timing of intercourse to the probability of conception and the sex of the baby." *Biometrics* 50: 358-367.

Wilcox, A.J., Weinberg, C.R. et al. 1995. "Timing of sexual intercourse in relation to ovulation. Effects on probability of conception, survival of the pregnancy, and sex of baby." *New England Journal of Medicine* 333 (23): 1517-1521.

Wilcox, A.J., Weinberg, C.R. et al. 1988. "Incidence of early loss of pregnancy." *New England Journal of Medicine* 319 (4): 189-194.

———. 1985. "Measuring early pregnancy loss: laboratory and field methods." *Fertility and Sterility* 44 (3): 366-74.

World Health Organization. 1981. "A prospective multi-centre trial of the ovulation method of natural family planning. I. The teaching phase." *Fertility & Sterility* 36 (2) Aug: 152-158.

Yuzpe, A., L. Z. Albert, et al. 2000. "Rescue intracytoplasmic sperm injection (ICSI)- salvaging in vitro fertilization (IVF) cycles after total or near-total fertilization failure." *Fertility & Sterility* 73: 1115-1119.

Zhou, H. and C. Weinberg. 1996. "Modeling conception as an aggregated Bernoulli outcome with latent variables, via the EM algorithm." *Biometrics* 52: 945-954.

Zhou, H., C. Weinberg, et al. 1996. "A random-effects model for cycle viability in fertility studies." *Journal of American Statistical Association* 91: 1413-1422.

Perimenopause: Physiological Parameters
Nancy Reame, Ph.D., R.N.
Professor - University of Michigan

Professor Nancy Reame presented physiological reasons for the decline of fertility among peri-menopausal women. Her presentation included a description of a new consensus model and definition for the process of peri-menopause. The model represents an executive summary from the Stages of Reproductive Aging Workshop in which she participated. Called the STRAW staging system, the paper "Executive summary: Stages of Reproductive Aging Workshop (STRAW)" has been reproduced for this proceedings book at the request of Dr. Reame and with permission from the publisher Elsevier Science and the American Society for Reproductive Medicine (Fertility and Sterility, 2001, 76, pp 874-78.). Please see Appendix 1 of these proceedings book for a reprint of this article.

Perimenopause
Respondent:
Kathleen M. Raviele, M.D., F.A.C.O.G.

The years of the perimenopause, defined as the period immediately preceding and following menopause, can be some of the most challenging for couples using Natural Family Planning. For many women it is concern over achieving a pregnancy late in their reproductive lives, with concern for congenital abnormalities or health problems. For others who either waited until their late 30s to start a family, or married late or had a change of heart about contraception or sterilization, it is infertility.

Menopause is gradual and first presents with subtle symptoms. Ninety percent of women have irregular cycles for up to four years before they cease. The median age is 51, but 2% of women will have permanent cessation of menses under the age of 40 (Novak 1996, 981-982). There is a decline in fecundability, or the ability to conceive, as women age. This appears to be primarily related to the aging of a woman's oocytes. In oocyte donor programs where older women conceive by in vitro with a younger woman's oocytes, the pregnancy rates are the same as for younger women (Johnson 2000, 70). Thus, the primary cause of reproductive failure in older women is diminished ovarian reserve with loss of oocytes and decreased responsiveness to gonadotropins. (Scott 1995, 1-11)

In human females, the oogonia complete their proliferative phase during fetal life and enter meiosis in the first meiotic prophase where they arrest as primordial oocytes in primordial follicles. They may stay in this arrested phase for up to 50 years. A large number of follicles die off around the time of birth, but at menarche, a continuous stream of follicles recommence growth each day. These follicles pass through three stages of growth: the primary or preantral follicle; the secondary or antral follicle; then finally a preovulatory follicle. The time table to do this varies with the preovulatory phase being the shortest. The preantral follicle experiences oocyte growth, granulosa cell proliferation and follicular growth. This growth appears to be independent of extraovarian control, perhaps under the influence of growth factors within the ovary. The theca cells develop which bind LH and synthesize androgens from acetate and cholesterol, stimulated by LH. The granulosa cells bind FSH and produce 17B estradiol and estrone from aromatization of thecal androgens called cell co-cooperation, and de novo synthesis from acetate in thecal cells.

The late preantral and early antral follicles become atretic if not exposed to tonic levels of FSH and LH and the expanding antral follicle dies unless there is a brief surge of LH. This results in ovulation and conversion of the follicle into the corpus luteum (Johnson 2000, 70-77).

Women's peak fertility is at age 25. There is an initial drop in fertility at age 32, a sharper drop at age 35, followed by a precipitous drop at age 40. Ninety-four percent of women can conceive before the age of 25, 57% between the ages of 36–40, and only 25% of women between the ages of 40–45. They are usually women who have already had children, and pregnancy is rare after the age of 45. The reason appears to be increased failed ovulations, increased miscarriages and increased perinatal and neonatal abnormality (Scott 1995, 1-11).

As the oocytes age, having been suspended in first meiotic prophase for 35+ years, they show increased meoitic spindle instability and chromosomal changes. Ovarian dispersium follicles become increasingly resistant to FSH but estradiol levels may remain constant. Blood work may show a normal estradiol level in a woman having hot flashes or night sweats. The rise in FSH is caused by a decline in ovarian inhibin factor.

Inhibins are a class of proteins made by the granulosa cells in late antral phase and the corpus luteum of the follicle and they play a role in the negative feedback regulation of FSH. Inhibin B is decreased early in the menstrual cycle in a perimenopausal woman causing a rise in FSH. The initial rise in FSH will cause an increase in estrogen levels, perhaps higher than what is seen in younger women. This coupled with anovulatory cycles, may cause increased mucus. Estradiol levels may remain normal until a few years before menopause (Johnson 2000, 96-98). After ovulation, the corpus luteum produces inhibin A, and this also decreases as menopause approaches, raising FSH levels.

The onset of symptoms of menopause include: mood changes, irritability, loss of libido, hot flashes, night sweats, vaginal dryness, mental confusion, memory loss, insomnia and shrinkage of the reproductive organs, together with irregular cycles. These symptoms may precede menopause, defined as the absence of a period for one year with cessation of ovarian activity, by several years.

If an older woman is trying to achieve a pregnancy, how can we determine if she has adequate ovarian reserve? Classically, it is recommended to do a baseline FSH level on day 3 of the cycle. If it is greater than 15 miu/ml, she is not likely to respond to ovulation induction. If it is greater that 25 miu/ml, even if she achieves a pregnancy, the miscarriage rate is high, and if it is 30 mu/ml or greater, textbooks state the woman no longer has to worry about pregnancy (Scott 1989, 651-654).

Here are the results of 3 patients from my practice:

Patient A: Age 41, G3P3, hot flashes irregular cycles, FSH 30.9
   Age 42, three months amenorrhea, FSH 52.1, Estradiol 76
   Withdrawal period after Provera
   Conceived the next cycle, elective abortion
   Had last menses four months later

Patient B: Age 41, G7P4, menopausal symptoms, no skipped menses. FSH 16.5 on menses, estradiol 35, conceived next cycle

Patient C: Age 44, G5P5 irregular cycles
Age 47, serial FSH levels on menses - 51.0, 115.4, 40.5, 32.7
Endometrial biopsy showed complex glandular hyperplasia, given cyclic progesterone
   Age 48, FSH 9.3, 70.3, still seeing lots of mucus
   Age 51, still having sporadic light menses

As you can see, ovarian function is unique for each individual. In addition to doing day 3 FSH levels, the Clomiphene Challenge Test was proposed for infertility couples over the age of 30 in 1987 by Navot et al. A baseline FSH level is done day 3, Clomid 100 mg is given days 5-9 and a repeat FSH level is done on day 10. Women who have a normal ovarian reserve will be able to suppress the FSH level by day 10. Normal levels are FSH 3 + FSH 10 <26 miu/ml. An abnormal CCT shows poor reproductive performance regardless of age, but over the age of 40, a normal CCT still does not indicate a woman will be able to get pregnant as she may have already experienced a significant depletion of oocytes (Scott 1993, 539-543).

In summary, menopause is a natural event and is part of aging in women. As we teach couples NFP, it is helpful to share with older couples the natural decline in fecundability that women experience after the age of 32, so they can make an informed choice on when to start a family. We also can be reassuring to women trying to avoid pregnancy after the age of 45 that the chances of pregnancy are low, even without natural family planning. In addition, couples who seek to learn natural family planning for infertility and are older can have more realistic expectations of their success depending on the woman's ovarian reserve as determined at least by a basal FSH level on day 3. However, a woman of proven fecundity – ability to conceive and carry to term - who is under the age of 45 needs to follow the rules of her method of NFP if the couple wants to avoid pregnancy as there is no definite blood work that will confirm she is absolutely infertile until she has gone one year without a menses.

Kathleen Raviele, M.D.
Obstetrics and Gynecology
Atlanta, GA

Bibliography

Berek, J. 1996. *Novak's Gynecology.* Baltimore: Williams & Wilkins: 981-982.

Johnson, M., and Everitt, B. 2000. *Essential Reproduction.* Oxford: Blackwell Science Ltd: 70-77, 96-98.

Navot, D., Rosenwaks, Z., and Margalioth, E.J. 1987. "Prognostic assessments of female fecundity." *Lancet* ii:645-7.

Scott, R., Toner, J., Muasher, S., Oehninger, S., Robinson S., and Rosenwaks Z. 1989. "FSH levels on cycle day 3 are predictive of invitro fertilization outcome." *Fertility and Sterility* 5:651-654.

Scott, R., Leonardi, M., Hofmann, G., Innions, E., Neal, G., and Navot D. 1993. "A prospective evaluation of clomiphene citrate challenge test screening of the general infertility population." *Obstetrics and Gynecology* 83:539-45.

Scott, R., and Hofmann, G. 1995. "Prognostic assessment of ovarian reserve." *Fertility and Sterility* 63: 1-11.

Toner, J., Philput, C., Jones, G., and Muasher, S. 1991. "Basal FSH level is a better predictor of invitro fertilization performance than age." *Fertility and Sterility* 55:784-91.

Efficacy of a new method of family planning: the Standard Days Method
Marcos Arevalo, M.D., M.P.H.
Victoria Jennings, Ph.D.
Irit Sinai, Ph.D.
Georgetown University Institute for Reproductive Health

Marcos Arevalo, M.D., Assistant Professor and Director of Biomedical Research at the Georgetown University Institute for Reproductive Health presented a new fixed day calendar system of family planning called the Standard Day Method (SDM). Dr. Arevalo's paper (co-authored with Victoria Jennings, Ph.D., Professor and Director of the Institute and Irit Sinai, Ph.D., Assistant Professor and Senior Research Officer at the Institute) described the Cyclebead system used with the SDM and presented the results of an effectiveness study of the new method. At the request of Dr. Arevalo and with permission of Elsevier Science their paper "Efficacy of a new method of family planning: the Standard Days Method" was reprinted from the journal *Contraception*, 2001;65:333-338. See Appendix 2 of these proceedings book for a reprint of this article.

Response to Arevalo, Jennings, & Sinai's paper
"Efficacy of a new method of family planning: the Standard Days Method"
Joseph B. Stanford, M.D., M.S.P.H.

Consider two Natural Family Planning (NFP) method efficacy studies. One study is of a high-tech method based on urinary hormones. The other is of a simple calendar-based method. The method pregnancy rates are 4.8 and 6.2, and the typical use pregnancy rates are 12.0 and 29.2, respectively. Guess which one is which? The study with the higher pregnancy rates was the high-tech method (Persona) (Bonnar et al., 1999). The one with the lower pregnancy rates was a study of the Standard Days Method (Arevalo, Jennings, Sinai 2002). This should serve as a reminder that we should not be too quick to dismiss simple ideas, nor should we jump to the idea that more technology is always better.

This study had a number of strengths. It was a "model" effectiveness study in terms of enrollment, design, execution, and statistical analysis. The denominators were calculated correctly for the method-related and typical-use pregnancy rates. We can be confident of the results for the populations studied.

As a parenthetical note, this study provides some important insight into the use of barrier methods at the fertile time, an important and sometimes controversial issue in NFP. Some studies have suggested higher pregnancy rates from the use of barriers at the fertile time (as opposed to abstinence), while others have not. This study found that couples who used barriers or withdrawal during the fertile time had a method pregnancy rate of 5.7, whereas couples who abstained during the fertile time had a pregnancy rate of 4.8. Given the methodologic strengths of this study, this is the best estimate we have to date of the "real" effect of barriers or withdrawal during the fertile time. It makes sense that the pregnancy rates should be a little higher for such behavior, and this study confirms that.

This leads to the main weakness of this study, and the major weakness of the Standard Days Method. Not all women can use it. In fact, many women at any given time cannot use it, and almost all women will not be able to use it at some point of their reproductive lives, because of the requirement that women generally have cycles between 26-32 days. Unfortunately, we do not know how many women applied to be in the study but were excluded based on these criteria. What we do know is that 28% of women who were found eligible for the study had to be withdrawn from the study because they had two cycles that fell out of the required range during follow-up. This method meets the need of only a minority of women of reproductive age.

It is of great significance that those who had to be withdrawn from the study because of two cycles being out of range chose to continue using the Standard Days Method, even though they were told that its effectiveness in this situation would be significantly less. This shows how hungry couples in developing countries are for natural methods. This method fills a real need, but unfortunately it does so only incompletely.

The Standard Days Method is not as effective as other modern methods of NFP, such as the Billings Method, the Creighton Model FertilityCare™ System, or the Sympto-Thermal Method. Any one of these methods would be more likely to meet the needs of a wide spectrum of couples, with cycles of different lengths, in different reproductive categories. In particular, the Billings Method has a long distinguished track record of meeting the needs of many couples in many developing countries.

However, the Standard Days Method may be able to be immediately accessible to couples where other established NFP methods may take years to train teachers and to develop infrastructure, not to mention to address the essential need for respectful and collaborative relationships with governmental and public family planning agencies. The Standard Days Method can be disseminated much more rapidly and easily. The same might be true of the Two Day Method, still in development, also from Georgetown University. In many areas, all that is offered to couples are pills, IUDs, and sterilization, or nothing at all. The need is desperate and immediate for a natural method worldwide, and many couples are hungry for a natural method, whether they know it or not.

If the introduction of the Standard Days Method leads to a rapid increase of couples that are able to use natural method worldwide; and also leads to the subsequent introduction and acceptance of other natural methods that can meet the needs of those who don't fit the criteria for the Standard Days Method, then all the effort that went into the development and dissemination of the Standard Days Method will have been worth it.

Bibliography

Bonnar, J., Flynn, A. et al. 1999. "Personal hormone monitoring for contraception." *British Journal of Family Planning* 24:128-134.

Arevalo, M., Jennings, V., and Sinai, I. 2002. "Efficacy of a new method of family planning: the Standard Days Method." *Contraception* 65:333-338.

Psychological Aspects of Achieving or Avoiding Pregnancy

Lawrence J. Severy
The R. David Thomas Professor of Psychology, University of Florida & Director, Behavioral and Social Sciences, Family Health International

and

Janet Robinson
Family Health International

Both the creation of a child, and the alternative, the avoidance and prevention of an unwanted pregnancy, reflect complex processes involving two individuals. For the psychologist there are two phenomena of interest. First, there are the individual values, desires, intentions, and actions relating to either proception or contraception. And, second, there are the interpersonal processes engaged in wherein these two perspectives are blended so as to result in joint decisions and joint courses of action. As Marie Harvey from the University of Oregon and the Pacific Women's Health Group likes to say, there is an old Sufi saying that "you think you understand two because you understand *one* and *one*... But you must also understand *and*" (Harvey 2001). Social scientists are just now beginning to delineate the ways in which couples operationalize "and." The purpose of this paper is to review some of the ideas and data related to the acceptability of methods, especially the new methods that couples employ while seeking to conceive or contracept.

Acceptability–A Conceptual Analysis

The concept of finding something "acceptable" is clearly an individual level construct. The vast majority of method "acceptability" research papers delineate the way in which men or women (sometimes both) respond to the features of the product being rated. And, often, a single score is generated to reflect the "overall" acceptability rating. To the psychologist, to say that something is *acceptable* implies some aspects of an evaluation or judgment, but not others. If something is thought to be acceptable, we do not even know that the product is liked. Acceptability may simply convey we will not go out of our way to avoid or prevent product use. Further, although we might find something acceptable, it does not imply that we might we try it. The further clarification of these opinions probably depends upon whether there is an alternative option that we find even more, or less, acceptable.

Perhaps a more useful term would be "*prefer*" or to say that one product or method is "preferable" to another. In this case, we have what amounts to a rank ordering of approaches. That said, we might prefer the better of two absolutely terrific options, or we might prefer the best of two extremely unattractive alternatives. We often label this later case an instance of choosing the least bad alternative—something I often find myself doing on election day.

When it is the case that the two alternatives are bad, and yet that we must choose one, the term most likely used is "tolerate." For example, we are willing to tolerate the lesser of two evils. When it comes to proception or contraception, it is likely the case that most people would prefer to use absolutely nothing. However, they often find themselves in need of assistance, choosing a method that they can tolerate, if not actually like.

These three terms allow us to understand seemingly illogical behavior. Why would someone not use a method to assist with proception or contraception if they really liked the method? Clearly, they liked something else better, i.e., they preferred a second approach. Conversely, why would someone persist in using something that they did not like? Obviously, they do not like any of the options, and although they would prefer to not use anything, they are willing to tolerate the least offensive option.

As argued by Ian Askew (1994), "research that examines the acceptability of family planning technologies has played an important role within the broader scheme of developing effective family planning program structures and processes" since the 1970's. Cleland, Hardy and Taucher (1990) identified three different types of such acceptability research. These types are still relevant, although we might expand and enhance their descriptions. These researchers talked about "hypothetical acceptability," "initial acceptability" and "experiential acceptability." The first of these, hypothetical acceptability, is often studied prior to the development of a product. The potential developer or manufacturer is interested in knowing what the market segment of market share might be for such a product. Market segment refers to the identification of who might be interested, and market share is designed to capture the prevalence of interest. Often, developers are interested in what might be perceived to be the attractive or unattractive features of a hypothetical product—features that could be added or avoided as they develop their product or program concepts. In fact, hypothetical acceptability is clearly most dependent upon ratings of potential product features. Last but not least, developers would love to know how much someone would be willing to pay for their new product. This is not a trivial issue as it can be argued that by the time new products make their way through required clinical trials, costs typically exceed more than 100 million dollars per innovation.

For Cleland et al. (1990) the term initial acceptability reflected a "willingness to try" something. Note that a willingness does not really imply that one actually does try, only that you are willing to try. Perhaps what is needed is an acknowledgement that one actually does try, if even for a brief time period. Even though we might label this short-term acceptability, it is important. Marketers often inundate us with "free samples" with the goal being to entice us to try a new product. Clearly, they believe that once having tried a product, we will continue to buy and use it. In behavioral change models (Prochaska and DiClemente 1994) it might be argued that acceptability at this stage implies that the potential user has performed two steps—first they have decided that they may be in need of the product (labeling) and second that they are committed to try. As Minnis and Padian (2001) suggest, this stage might be termed the "choice" stage. In other words, even though you have not yet used the product, you think you should and have decided that among alternatives, this is the correct approach. Unfortunately for marketers and those favoring the "free sample" procedure, Minnis and Padian (2001) find extremely little evidence that "choice" successfully predicts actual use, and/or use over time.

The last term in the Cleland et al. framework is "experiential" acceptability. They mean that after having used (experienced) the method, people will either come to like it or not, use it correctly and consistently or not. Again in the marketing genre, the term product "satisfaction" might be more typically employed. As for behavioral change models, the transition is from commitment to "enactment." Behavioral change modelers somewhat parallel the distinctions made among the terms: attitudes, behavioral intentions and behavior.

The term that is missing in the three-fold framework, but present in the behavioral change approach, is "maintenance." The important point here is that even though people may try something for awhile, even though it is very good for them (such as heart medicines) people regress to earlier stages and simply are not consistent users of products and methods. For example, the complaints regarding the effectiveness of condoms surrounds the issue of the requirement that they must be used correctly and consistently—something humans often have trouble with. The type of acceptability that is most important to the purposes of this paper is this last type of acceptability—sustained and correct use over time.

What is meant by "and"?

There is a growing body of scholarly literature documenting that obtaining data from both partners involved in proception and contraception decisions and activities surpasses explanations dependent upon only one of the partners—typically the woman. For example, Thomson and Hoem (1998) demonstrate that a woman's ratings, and ratings of what she believes to be true for her partner, do not serve as effective proxies for the man's actual ratings regarding different forms of contraception.

That said, the question becomes "What is the most productive and psychologically meaningful way in which to utilize both partners data in analyses of predicting fertility behavior, and acceptability studies of methods related to fertility regulating methods?" Amazingly, there are at least six different mathematical procedures that are possible, and each implies a different set of psychological assumptions about the nature of joint decision making regarding fertility issues (Miller, Severy and Pasta 2002).

First, in the most simplistic approach, both the female and male data are treated as independent variables in predictions of behavior. Statistically, the procedure involves entering all variables into a regression equation. Note that there is no real attempt to consider combining the data, or the extent of a potential mathematical relationship between the female and male data. The assumption here is that these are simply independent data points, with no requirement that the other partner be aware of, or ever have discussed, the partner's perspective. In fact, there may be no relationship!

Second, an obvious approach is to combine the male and female data on each variable by either totaling the two scores into a single score, or computing their average. Mathematically, these two options result in the same type of information. The assumption behind this procedure is that the two partners are equally important, and that the best way to represent the couple's feelings is to generate a single score derived from information provided by each.

Third, another way of combining the two data points is to subtract them. In this case we can tell about the degree of partner consensus, or the lack thereof. This is especially true if the difference score is treated as an absolute value. In this manner it is not important if the wife is more favorable than the husband, or vice versa. What does matter is whether they disagree by a small amount or a large amount. The fourth approach to combining the data would take note of whether the female or male is the most favorable. In this case the difference score would be an algebraic total. For example, by always subtracting the male score from the female score, positive differences would indicate that she is more favorable, while negative scores would indicate that the male is more favorable.

It is also important to note that difference scores are somewhat independent of the total or average score (the second approach). For example, disagreeing by one scale point does not indicate if the scale point difference is between "like" versus "very much like" on the favorable side, or "dislike" versus "very much dislike" on the negative side. The implication is that perhaps both degree of consensus *and* the total or average score need to be included as predictors of fertility related behavior.

The fifth and sixth approaches reflect yet again different psychological processes. There is evidence that it is often the most negative information that drives our decisions and attitudes. (People tend to minimize their maximum possible loss.) Therefore, one way to operationalize this possibility is to only use the most negative of the two partner's scores as the single score for the couple. The rationale is simply that at least one of the partners really does not like something, and that in discussions, this position, in essence, will veto any alternative position taken by the partner. The exact opposite strategy is to consider the most positive partner's position as the couple's score. The rationale for this index is that there is a true champion for the rating, and, again in discussions, this partner would influence the other and dominate the ratings.

Our position is that there is no one particular "correct" combination rule for handling couple data. Rather, each of these six approaches addresses slightly different issues and depends upon different underlying assumptions reflecting the couple decision making process. Depending upon the nature of the study, and the assumptions or questions being addressed, any one of the procedures may be the best one (or two) to use.

Couple acceptability of fertility regulating methods.

As presented above, Thomson and Hoem (1998) have demonstrated that factors associated with both partners help to explain contraceptive choice and use. Earlier, Severy and Silver (1993) had discovered that with many fertility regulation methods, input from the husband and wife were approximately equal in importance to the decision and use. Thomson (1997) has also noted that individuals often consider their own opinions when asked to report those of their partners. In other words, the perception of one's partner is modified by projections of one's own position. Thus, multiple findings suggest the value in asking both partners for their opinions and ratings when evaluating fertility regulating methods.

As might be imagined, the degree and quality of the communication activity demonstrated by a couple has an important impact on decision making and other behavior. Couple communication has been shown to help change sexual behavior (Tullman, Gilner, Kolodny, Dornbush and Tullman 1981) and facilitate the use of contraception (Polit-O'Hara and Kahn 1985). More recently, Catania and his colleagues have found that those individuals who are best able to communicate their desire for "safer sex," ask about their partner's prior sexual history, and share their own experiences, are the most likely to use condoms successfully (Catania, Coates, Golden and Dolcini 1994). This may be another way of saying that those who are open with their partners, and sufficiently self assured, are more likely to demonstrate high quality communication. An interesting twist on these findings is reported by Severy and Silver (1993). They found that husbands were almost twice as successful as their wives in accurately predicting their partner's beliefs regarding an array of contraceptive alternatives. Their interpretation was that women were more likely to talk about their opinions, hence making it possible for the men to accurately report their wives' opinions. The reverse was probably not true, and with men being relatively non-communicative, the women were forced to guess.

In addition to communication factors, another domain demanding increasing attention is the potential impact of the method on the intimate relationship enjoyed by the partners. The potential impact on sexual pleasure was the main reason given by Mexican women in their evaluation of new methods involving gels or creams (Garcia et al, 1997). Severy and Spieler (2000) argue that the prospect of enhancing sexual pleasure should be a driving force and feature of new methods, if developers wish to succeed with new products. There is some evidence that methods can increase pleasure (Bentley 2000; Pool et al. 2000), in this case with proxies for currently in development microbicides. Further, sexual pleasure and self-esteem were the two most important predictors of condom use in a recent study of 4,000 U.S. women (Albarracin et al. 2000). Clearly, the impact on sexual enjoyment must be monitored in studies of new method acceptability.

Historically, data were only collected from women as it was thought that "women are responsible for that sort of thing." In some cultures, Woodsong (2002) still finds that men prefer "women initiated" methods as it "lets them [men] off the hook" regarding responsibility. On the other hand, there are data suggesting that when men supervise their wives behavior, women's behavior is more consistent and effective. For example, Deys and Potts (1975) found that among Iranian women, effective pill-taking rose from 12 to 93 percent when the husband was involved. And, in male-dominated Ethiopia, having men participate in family planning home visits increased the use of modern methods (Terefe and Larson 1993). Aral (1992), of the CDC, has suggested that in settings wherein women lack power in interpersonal relationship, it is imperative to focus on programming for men. Hence the nature of the overall relationship being expressed by the couple is extremely important.

PERSONA acceptability trials– The United Kingdom

The above distinctions and identified important parameters help define the elements of a comprehensive investigation of the acceptability of new fertility related methods. More specifically, the remainder of this paper is devoted to a review of two types of products - a device designed to assist couples trying to avoid a pregnancy, and a device designed to assist couples achieve a desired pregnancy. Both products were developed by the Unipath Diagnostics Company, and are for sale in some (mostly European) countries. Both products depend upon the home monitoring of LH and E3G in a woman's morning urine. More information regarding the exact process is available from Unipath, and the report of the contraceptive efficacy of PERSONA is reported by Bonnar, Flynn, Freundl, Kirkman, Roystan and Snowden (1999). Our presentation starts with a description of trials conducted both in the United Kingdom and the United States addressing the acceptability of PERSONA. Subsequently, the description of a U.S. based acceptability trial of the Clearplan Easy Fertility Monitor will be presented.

As described by Bonnar et al, the PERSONA efficacy trials in Europe involved 710 women and their partners. Couples were recruited from the general population in England, Ireland and Germany. Acceptability data were collected from only the subset of English women and their partners by Robert Snowden and his associates at the Institute for Population Studies, University of Exeter, Devon, England. These data were reported by Severy, et al (2002) and are briefly reviewed here. In order to qualify for the study, women were required to: be between the ages of 18 and 45; have regular menstrual cycles; be sexually active; be devoid of infertility problems; commit to being in the study for at least 12 months; have not used hormonal methods within the last

Psychological Aspects of Achieving or Avoiding Pregnancy 119

three months; and have had at least three months since the return of menses after pregnancy.

The English study obtained information from the partners after the first, sixth and twelfth menstrual cycles. In essence, the assessment of acceptability focused upon: overall levels of acceptance, ratings of the features and required procedures, trust in the information, and the quality of the couple relationship. To start, women reported that using PERSONA was simple and direct. As is depicted in Figure 1, the vast majority of trial participants quickly learned and accepted the required procedures.

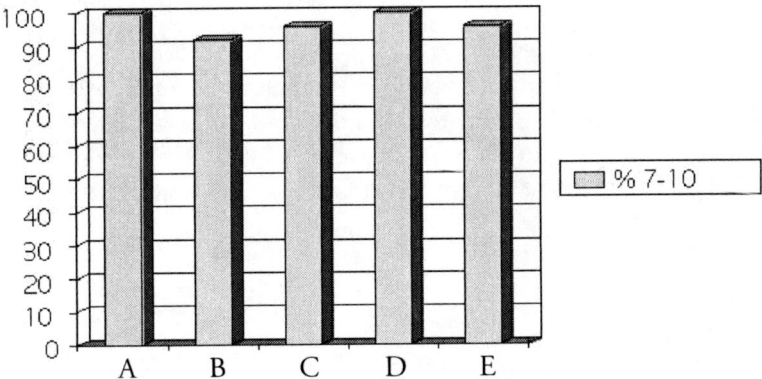

Figure 1. Percent of volunteers rating ease of use (at least 7 on a 10 point scale) as (A) resetting each cycle, (B) looking at daily, (C) using test stick, (D) understanding result, and (E) understanding instruction booklet.

PERSONA identifies both the days during which conception might be possible (red lights) as well as the days during which conception is highly unlikely (green lights). English women rated how well they trusted the information regarding the red and green light days. As can be seen in Figure 2, these ratings of trust increase over time. And, they are more willing to believe, or they are more motivated to believe, the green lights. Note that trust in the red lights increases only after the algorithm individuates to the woman's own bodily functioning after the fourth cycle.

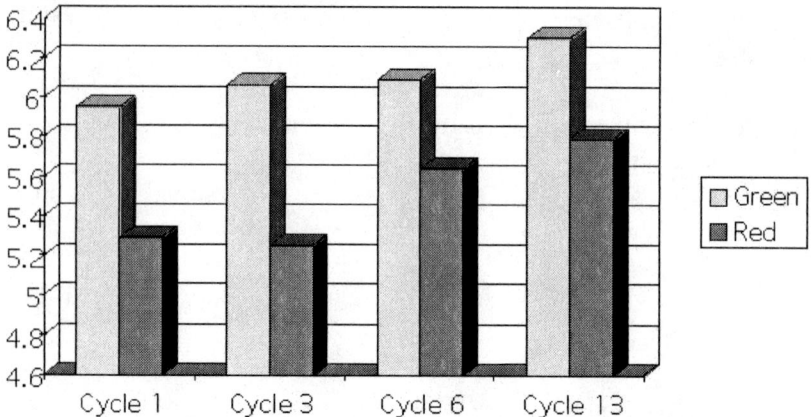

Figure 2. Perceived accuracy of green and red lights.

The impact on intimate relations at the end of six months is depicted in Figure 3. Clearly, there are only a very few couples who report that aspect of their relationship getting worse. The vast majority report no change, or that their sex life is even better while using PERSONA.

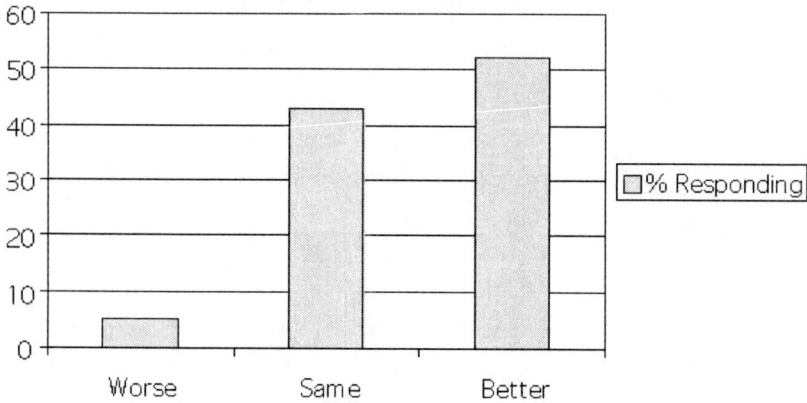

Figure 3. Percent responding to query, "since using the monitor my sex life is ...." Date obtained after six cycles of use.

As for an overall evaluation, acceptability was somewhat dependent upon other factors. More specifically, no one method of fertility control is going to be the answer for each and every couple. Some couples will prefer methods not at all liked by others. In the case of PERSONA, as rated by the English women, acceptability was related to the number of children in the family at the time of the method use. As is shown in Figure 4, trust in the monitor decreases with increasing family size. These couples probably are adverse to any future family building. In such cases, couples want a method with even higher claims regarding efficacy. Those most trusting raters were those couples with only one child, perhaps not dedicated to avoid any and all future pregnancies. Such couples are probably spacing their children and use a family planning method to achieve their desired result.

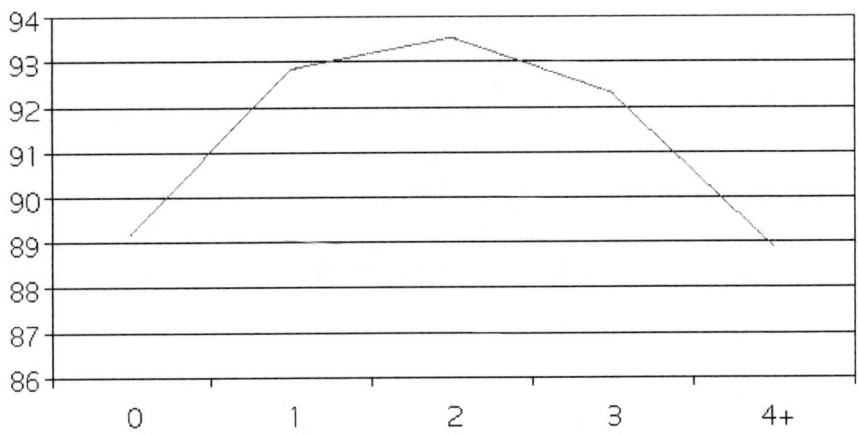

Figure 4. Mean trust ratings as a function of the number of children.

PERSONA acceptability trials–The United States

The US contraceptive efficacy trials upon which we piggybacked our studies of acceptability were conducted in California in the later half of the 1990s. Approximately 600 couples in the greater Los Angeles and San Francisco metropolitan areas were recruited to the study. One-half of the couples were randomly assigned to a control condition wherein they were to use condoms for fertility regulation during the one year long study. The other one-half of the couples were assigned to use the PERSONA monitor. Inclusion criteria for the women and their partners were the same as those delineated above for the European studies. The difference between the two trials was the use of a control group of couples in the U.S. studies.

Data were obtained independently from the clinical efficacy trials, and were mailed directly from the study participants to the principal investigator (Severy) at the University of Florida. It should also be noted that the female and male forms were also mailed separately so as to encourage total confidentiality—even from one's partner. Building and expanding upon the design of the English study, data were collected at baseline (after enrollment in the study but prior to the cycle beginning use of PERSONA), and after menstrual cycles 1,3,4,6 and 13. The reason for the 4th cycle assessment is that the monitor's algorithm changes between the third and fourth cycle—becoming more dependent upon the individual woman's bodily functioning. We wanted to assess the immediate impact of that modification. And, as some cycles are short, in order to complete a full calendar year, the end point was determined to be the 13th cycle.

The other important upgrade to the assessment of acceptability reflects the review and conceptual analysis presented earlier as an introduction to our empirical efforts. Data collected (N=418) during the baseline assessment allowed us to create scales reflective of the personal and interpersonal dimensions of acceptability. The statistical analyses utilized and the psychometric properties of these multidimensional scales are presented in Severy, McNulty, Klein and Jacobs (2002).

The acceptability scales and their respective estimates of reliability (*alphas*) are as follows:

- Overall acceptability of the method (.89)
- Confidence in the efficacy of the method (.75)
- One's perception of one's partner's degree of method acceptability (.77)
- Impact on the intimate relationship (.70)
- Impact on reproductive knowledge (.80)
- Overall quality of the couple's relationship (.75)
- Quality of partner communication (.86)
- Degree of self-efficacy/self-worth (.69)

All of these scales demonstrate at least statistically acceptable, if not, highly desirable reliability.

Also as reported by Severy et al. (2002), by using these scales at the inception of the study, it was possible to identify three basic "types" of

Psychological Aspects of Achieving or Avoiding Pregnancy

couples entering into the clinical trials. It is possible to briefly review the rather complex results of that (baseline) analysis. The fascinating finding is that after creation of the typology via cluster analytic techniques, we compared the final pregnancy rates for the three groups and found quite different results as a function of the couple's placement in the various groups. The first group of couples begs one to ask why they were in the study. They were in problematic relationships, did not think well of themselves, had the most kids, and were the most committed to not having another child. They did much better with condoms in comparison with PERSONA. The point is that PERSONA depends upon, and enhances relationship communication. These folks probably had little communication of a positive nature. The second group of couples really did not like their previous method, had been together for a shorter time frame, really liked each other, and were not adverse to having more children. They performed better with PERSONA in avoiding an unwanted pregnancy. The third, and largest, group scored the highest on all acceptability measures, and were the most likely to want more children in the future. Women in this group avoided unwanted pregnancy using either method better than women in the other groups, especially so when using PERSONA. So, it was only the troubled group that experienced fewer unwanted pregnancies with the use of condoms. Note that this is the only group with troublesome relationships.

The larger question is "what trends in acceptability occurred over time as a function of differential method use?" We present the results related to overall acceptability, impact on reproductive knowledge and impact on the intimate relationship here for the first time. Specifically, Figure 5 demonstrates the relative comparability of the two method groups at the baseline measure followed by the significantly more positive ratings for PERSONA over the next year. And, it is clear that although there is a little cyclical variation, acceptability increases over time, with the highest rating occurring at the 13th cycle. Ratings for use of the condom finish at almost exactly the same point as they started (at baseline).

What the monitor provides the user is clear identification of the stages of the woman's cycle. It would seem obvious that when asked, moni-

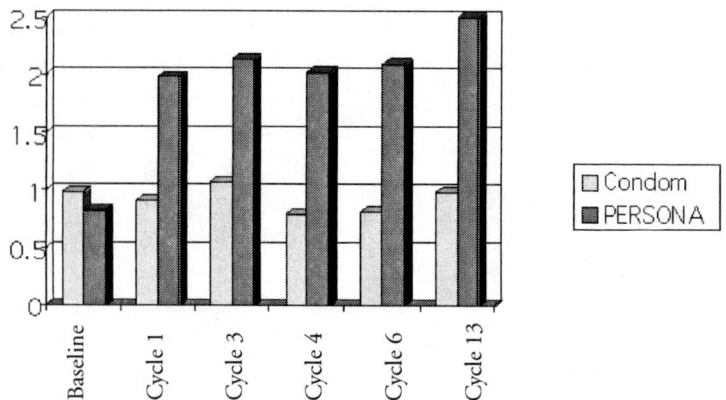

Figure 5. Overall acceptability of PERSONA versus condoms, over one year's experience of using.

tor users should report learning a lot more about their reproductive functioning in comparison to condom users. Figure 6 demonstrates this finding. Of interest is the fact that this increase in knowledge does not diminish over time, in fact the ratings again appear to increase.

One of the compelling arguments offered by supporters of Natural Family Planning is that use of the method might enhance couple communication. Figure 7 compares the reported impact on partner communication over the course of one year for monitor and condom using couples. Although there is again a cyclical trend, the fact is that

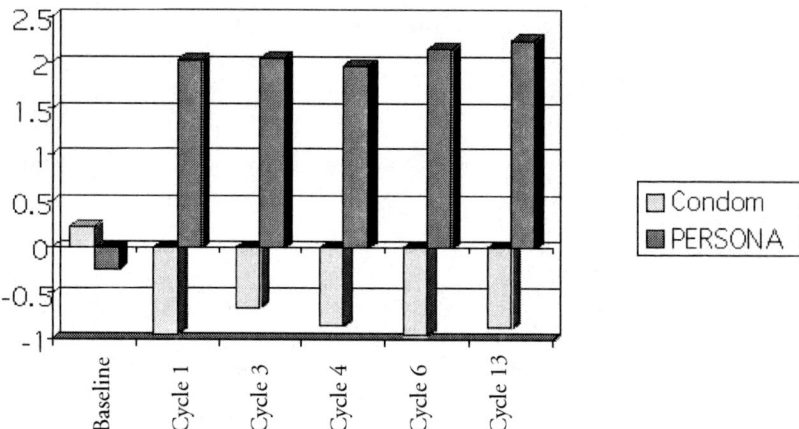

Figure 6. Impact on knowledge regarding reproductive functioning, over one year.

there is almost no difference between the two groups. It just may be that the assessment of this quality of couple relationship suffers from a "ceiling effect" or that the scale is too general in its scope or focus. At any rate, it is simply not the case that monitor use dramatically

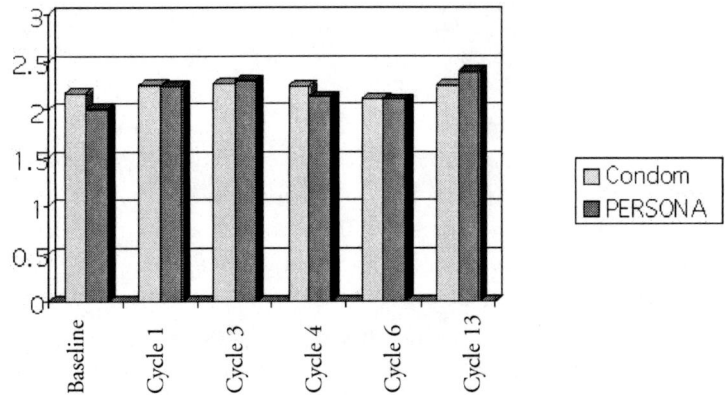

Figure 7. Impact on partner communication over one year.

impacts couple ratings in all dimensions. This finding actually enhances the interpretation of the earlier two results.

Clearplan Easy Fertility Monitor acceptability trials —The United States.

It did not take long for women to recognize the ability of PERSONA to inform them of the time during which they might get pregnant, and, therefore, perhaps the device might be useful to those trying, with some difficulty, to conceive. In turn, Unipath recognized that a meaningful proportion of the European PERSONA buyers were interested in this "off-label" purpose. Unipath also knew that although PERSONA targeted a range of days during which pregnancy was possible, PERSONA did not aggressively identify the days during which a conception was the very most likely to occur. Consequently, they developed a new monitor with a modified algorithm (the Clearplan Easy Fertility Monitor) which is designed to inform the woman and her partner about their prospects on any day. Specifically, the monitor contains a bar graph indicating that chances on the day in question are low, high or peak. Further, a symbol also identifies the day of ovulation.

The first trial of this proception monitor was conducted by Severy in conjunction with Pouru Bhiwandi in Raleigh, North Carolina, and Stan Williams in Gainesville, Florida. The efficacy results are presented elsewhere (Bhiwandi, Williams, Severy & Jacobs, 2001). However, suffice it to say that results were better than most assisted reproductive technology procedures. The study involved 60 couples, and acceptability data were also collected from both partners. These data are presented in Severy, Jacobs, Findley-Klein and McNulty (2002).

In order to monitor the acceptability of the Clearblue Easy Fertility Monitor, we developed a few new scales to compliment those used in the US PERSONA acceptability trials. Specifically, we were especially interested in scales that might tap the ebb and flow of stress, blame, and responsibility for success or failure in achieving a pregnancy. Therefore, additional dimensions monitored included: expectations of pregnancy success, sadness as a result of failing to achieve a pregnancy, sense of loss as a result of failing to achieve a pregnancy, and relationship strain. The mean *alpha* of these new scales was .90.

Given the data storage capabilities of these monitors, in conjunction with the acceptability questionnaires, and participants' diaries, it is possible to plot the cycle by cycle experiences of each couple. And, although all women in the study had the same goal—achieve a pregnancy, different patterns of behavior are displayed. One of the first questions that can be asked is whether couples utilize the information provided by the monitor to maximize their prospects for success. As Figure 8 depicts, couples clearly "target" their episodes of intercourse as a function of what the monitor is displaying. Whereas intercourse occurred on only 20% of the "low" fertility days (as displayed by the monitor), intercourse on "peak" days was experienced over 60% of the days. And, as is shown in Figure 9, this targeting of intercourse on "high" or "peak" days becomes much more dramatic over the four cycles of the study. Our assumption is that couple communication and strategizing became more deliberate as the study proceeded.

These data are rather complex as it is the case that at each cycle the number of couples remaining is diminished by the number of couples successfully achieving a pregnancy. Consequently, trends in acceptability scores over time as depicted in Figure 10 can be expected. Namely, those remaining at each data point tend to be a little less hopeful that

Psychological Aspects of Achieving or Avoiding Pregnancy

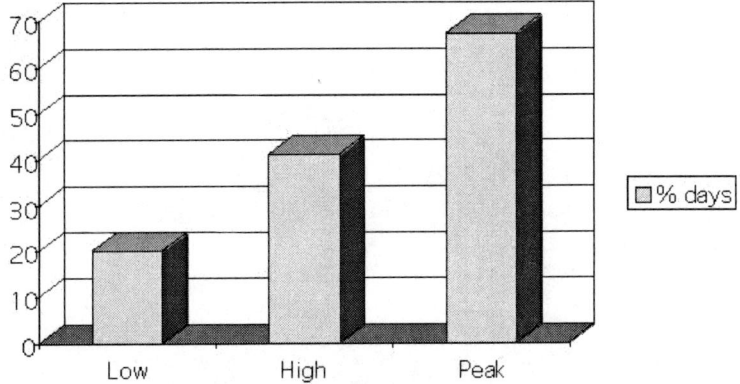

Figure 8. Sexual activity as a function of monitor status (% days of intercourse).

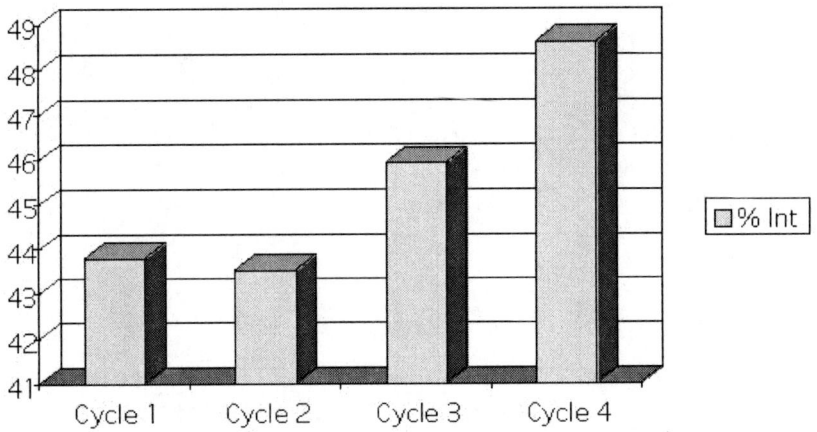

Figure 9. High plus peak monitor status sexual activity over 4 cycles.

those remaining at each previous time. And, in contradistinction, scores for relationship strain and blame, as well as anger and loss, tend to increase over time. That said, across the course of our study, levels of acceptability stayed very high, and anger/loss stayed low, with strain and blame remaining in the middle ranges.

One of the dimensions of special interest has always been the concern that a method of fertility regulation might actually serve a teaching function, allowing or informing the couple about the woman's reproductive functioning. As depicted in Figure 11, both males and females report "learning" from the monitor, with females consistently reporting higher scores. Further, this learning function clearly peaks at

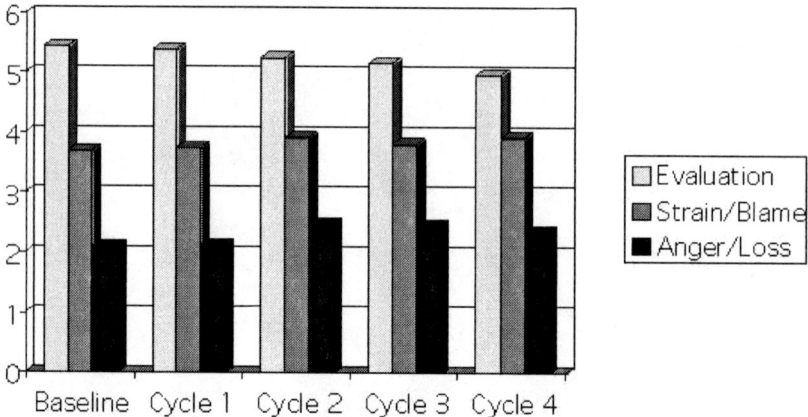

Figure 10. Evaluation, relationship strain and anger/loss over four cycles of use.

three (females) or four (males) cycles. If the study had been conducted for a longer period of time it would have been interesting to note if this downward trend continues.

A special variation on the above point is presented in Figure 12. Namely, note that at the end of each cycle we can determine which women became pregnant. Figure 12 presents the baseline data, collected

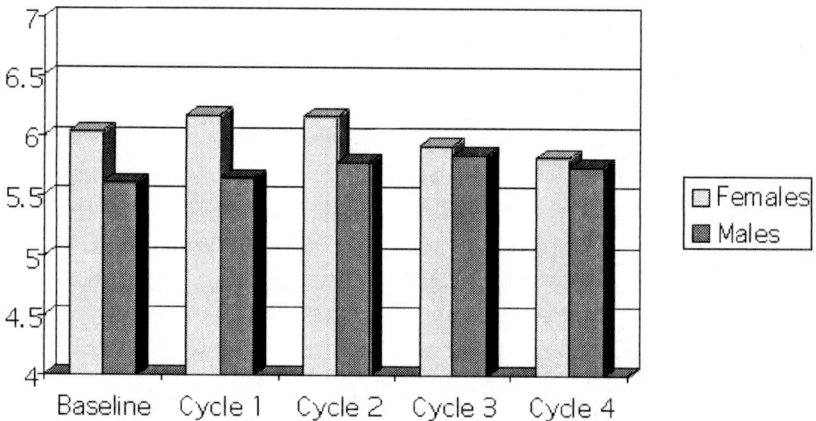

Figure 11. Effect on bodily functioning knowledge over 4 cycles.

prior to study inception. Note that in each case the group about to become pregnant during the study reported a higher level of acceptability and enthusiasm for the new monitor than those who were not successful. This seems to be a form of "self-fulfilling prophecy" and is quite dramatic. Implications are obvious, the monitor works best for those who think it will work! Figure 13 demonstrates the very

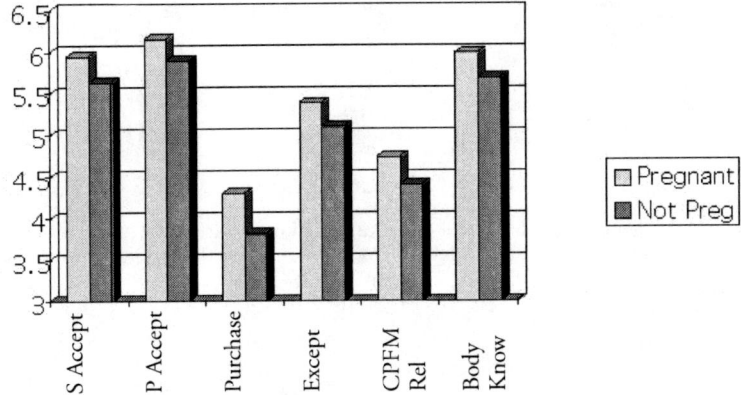

Figure 12. Baseline measure ratings by those couples that will become pregnant versus those who will not become pregnant.

different ratings by women regarding the knowledge function, and Figure 14 depicts the very different ratings of acceptability by the male partners.

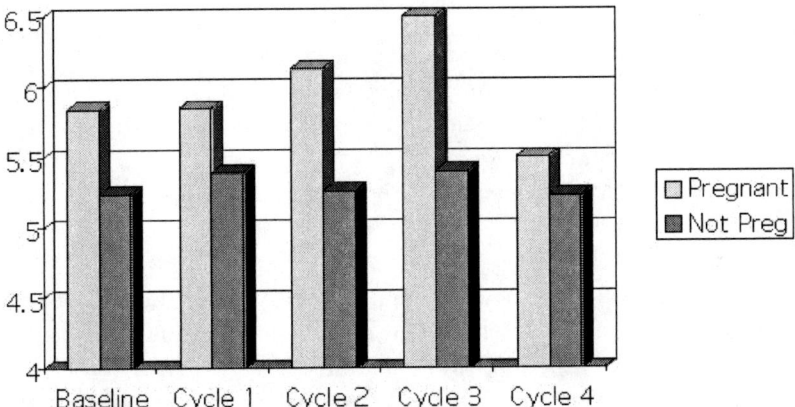

Figure 13. Male ratings of acceptability - Pregnant versus non-pregnant couples, as rated in the cycle prior to becoming pregnant.

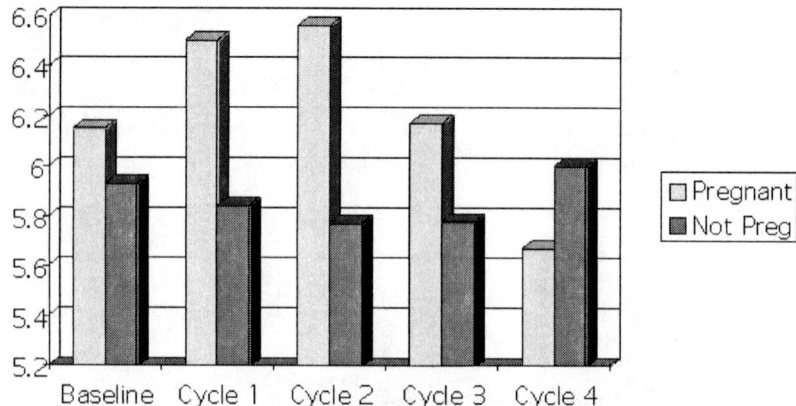

Figure 14. Female ratings of bodily function knowledge by pregnant versus non-pregnant couples, as rated in the cycle prior to becoming pregnant.

Summary and conclusions

It seems rather obvious to point out that couples would really rather not need to use anything when engaging in fertility and fertility regulating behavior. However, this is typically not the case. This paper actually starts with the premise that *if* something is needed, *if* something is to be used, what are the criteria for selection of that something? The conceptual distinctions and empirical results delineated here begin to provide us with a tentative response to what couples will accept, or at least tolerate. If something is to be used, couples seem to prefer:

a) non-invasive methods

b) methods that are as natural as they can be

c) methods that might actually serve an educational function, providing both partners with more information about the woman's reproductive functioning

d) methods that provide a positive impact on couple's communication and pleasure and

e) methods that work!

Another issue that deserves comment is whether the results over time are descriptive of what statisticians would formally characterize as a curvilinear function. In other words, is it the case that cycles of increasing acceptance and support eventually give way to decreasing enthusiasm? There are ways to interpret such a possibility. It may be that the initial enthusiasm simply reflects the excitement of experiencing something new, and whatever is new does not stay new over time. Interestingly, when we study the acceptability of well known methods the ratings typically depict a "flat line"—no growth and no decline. What is important to remember is that these choices, when something is needed, are truly unstable. People would really rather "not use" anything; therefore they are always looking for something better. As of now, the Unipath monitors seem to be the something better—but the prospect of another innovation is always around the corner. And, just because most couples enjoy these methods, there is no "one size fits all" product for fertility and fertility regulating behavior.

Bibliography

Albarricin, D., Ho, R., McNatt, P., Williams, W., Rhodes, F., Malotte, C.K., Hoxworth, T., Bolan, G., Zenilman, J. & Iatesta, M. 2000. "The structure of outcome beliefs in condom use." *Health Psychology* 19: 458-468.

Aral, S. 1992. "Sexual behavior as a risk factor for sexually transmitted disease." In A. Germain . Ed. *Reproductive tract infection.* New York: Plenum Press.

Askew, I. 1994. "Future directions for family planning operations research: Towards a greater appreciation of psychosocial issues." In L.J. Severy. Ed. *Advances in population: Psychosocial perspectives, Vol. 2.* London: Jessica Kingsley Publishers.

Bentley, M. 2000. "Acceptability of a novel vaginal microbicide, BufferGel, during a Phase I safety trial in Malawi, Zimbabwe, India and Thailand." Microbicides 2000 Conference. Alexandria, VA, March 13-16, 2000.

Bhiwandi, P.P., Williams, R.S., Severy, L.J. and Jacobs, J.E. 2001. "Assessment of the Clearplan Easy Fertility Monitor (CPFM) in couples seeking conception assistance." Meeting of the American College of Obstetrics and Gynecology.

Bonnar, J., Flynn, A., Freundl, G., Kirkman, R., Royston, R., and Snowden, R. 1999. "Personal hormone monitoring for contraception." *The British Journal of Family Planning* 24: 128-134.

Catania, J.A., Coates, T.J., Golden, E., Dolcini, M.M., Peterson, J., Kegeles, S., Siegel, D., and Fullilove, M.T. 1994. "Correlates of condom use among black, Hispanic, and white heterosexuals in San Francisco: The AIDS in Multi-Ethnic Neighborhoods survey." *AIDS Education Prevention* 6: 12-26.

Cleland, J., Hardy, E. and Taucher, E. 1990. *Introduction of new contraceptives into family planning programmes: Guidelines for social science research.* Geneva: World Health Organization.

Deys, C. and Potts, M. 1975. "Factors affecting patient motivation." In J. Sciarra, C. Markland, & J.J. Speidel. Eds. *Control of male fertility.* Hagerstown: Harper & Row.

Garcia, S., Snow, R. and Aitken, I. 1997. "Preferences for contraceptive attributes: Voices of women in Cuidad Juarez, Mexico." *International Family Planning Perspectives* 23: 52-58.

Harvey, S.M. 2001. "Preventing HIV/STDs and unintended pregnancy: A decade of challenges." Presented at the American Psychological Association meetings, San Francisco, August 26, 2001.

Miller, W.B., Severy, L.J. and Pasta, D.J. 2002. "Framework for modeling fertility motivation in the dyad." Submitted to *Personality and Social Psychology Review.*

Minnis, A.M. and Padian, N.S. 2001. "Does barrier contraceptive acceptability predict method use?" Presented at the American Psychological Association meetings, San Francisco, August 27, 2001.

Polit-O'Hara, D and Kahn, J.R. 1985. "Communication and contraceptive practices in adolescent couples." *Adolescence* 20: 33-43.

Pool, R., Whitworth, J., Green, G., Mbonye, A., Harrison, S., Hart, G., and Wilkinson, J. 2000. "Ambiguity, sexual pleasure, and the acceptability of microbicidal products in southwest Uganda." Microbicides 2000 Conference. Alexandria, VA, March 13-16, 2000.

Prochaska, J. O. and DiClemente, C.C. 1992. *Stages of Change in the Modification of Problem Behaviors.* Newbury Park, CA: Sage.

Severy, L.J. and Silver, S.E. 1993. "Two reasonable people: Joint decision-making in fefrtility regulation." In L.J. Severy. Ed. *Advances in population: Psychosocial perspectives, Vol.1* (pp. 207-227). London: Jessica Kingsley Publishers.

Severy, L.J. and Spieler, J. 2000. "New methods of family planning: Implications for intimate behavior." *Journal of Sex Research* 37: 258-265.

Severy, L.J., McNulty, J., Findley-Klein, F. and Jacobs, J. 2002. "Assessing the acceptability of innovative contraceptive technology: Participation profiles and implications for clinical trial success." Submitted to *Social Biology.*

Severy, L.J., Jacobs, J., Findley-Klein, C. and McNulty, J. "Psychosocial factors and couple dynamics in achieving a pregnancy with the aid of home monitoring: Assessing acceptability." Submitted to *Journal of Applied Social Psychology.*

Severy, L.J., Klein, C., and McNulty, J. 2002. "Acceptability of personal home monitoring for contraception: Longitudinal and contextual factors." *Journal of Social Psychology*. 142:87-96.

Terefe, A. and Larson, C. 1993. "Modern contraception use in Ethiopia: Does involving husbands make a difference?" *American Journal of Public Health* 83: 1567.

Thomson, E. 1997. "Couple childbearing desires, intentions, and births." *Demography* 34: 343-354.

Thomson, E. and Hoem, J. 1998. "Couple childbearing plans and births in Sweden." *Demography* 35: 315-322.

Tullman, G.M., Gilner, F.H., Kolodny, R.C., Dornbush, R.L., and Tullman, G.D. 1981. "The pre- and post-therapy measurement of communication skills of couples undergoing sex therapy at the Masters & Johnson Institute." *Archives of Sexual Behavior* 10: 95-109.

Response to paper by Lawrence Severy and Janet Robinson: "Psychological Aspects of Achieving or Avoiding Pregnancy"

Richard J. Fehring, D.N.Sc., R.N.
Professor, Marquette University

I read with great interest Severy and Robinson's paper on the psychological aspects of avoiding and achieving pregnancy. While reading and listening to the presentation I did so from both the perspective of teaching couples NFP and of researching the psycho-spiritual dynamics of practicing NFP. I found their paper and analysis refreshing because they provided a perspective that is new and unbiased to NFP. At the same time, many of the concepts in their paper are not new to NFP teachers and users from a sense that the information confirms what they (i.e., NFP teachers and users) already have experienced.

There is much to comment on in his paper, such as the dynamics and models of acceptability of new technology and new methods of family planning, the importance of communication and couple decision-making, the value of gaining reproductive knowledge and increased sexual intimacy with methods of family planning, how use of methods of family planning are enhanced through husband or male support, and how couples respond to the use of technology that aids in understanding the best time to achieve a pregnancy. Like Severy and Robinson, NFP teachers have noticed the differences and dynamics among what we call "limiters" and "spacers" in using a NFP method and how NFP does not work well when couples are having difficulties in their relationships. As teachers of NFP we also have experienced the various dynamics of couples trying to achieve pregnancies when they have infertility problems.

NFP teachers and advocates believe that NFP is "THE" ideal method of family planning and that NFP contributes to reproductive knowledge, enhances communication, intimacy, self-control, shared responsibility and shared decision-making and all of this without any medical side effects. And I believe that there is some evidence to support this. For example a recent study comparing oral contraceptives, sterilization, IUDs, condoms and NFP among German women showed that NFP was only second to sterilization in the ranking of sexual pleasure and first in regard to increased sexual desire (Oddens 1999). Furthermore, in a study I recently completed among current users of NFP almost 99% of the female users indicated that NFP increased their reproductive knowledge.

I was very excited by two content areas that I would call important gains of knowledge for NFP in Severy and Robinson's paper. The first is the development of a reliable scale for acceptability of family planning methods. The second is the tracking of psychological variables across time among users of a natural method of family planning, and the random comparison of these variables with a control group of couples using condoms. I will comment briefly on these two areas.

Through his research with users of Persona and the Clearplan Easy Fertility Monitor Dr. Severy has developed an acceptability tool that not only measures "acceptability" and "confidence of use" but also subscale measures of "partner communication," "reproductive knowledge," "intimacy," and "self-worth." These are all characteristics that NFP advocates claim the use of NFP will enhance in a marital relationship. We need more evidence that this is so and we need this evidence across time and in comparison with groups using different methods of family planning. And I would add with valid, reliable, and acceptable measurement tools. Having a standardized tool that could be utilized so that comparisons could be made with more confidence is a need in the area of NFP and family planning in general. I would like to know from Dr. Severy if he thinks that his tool could be adapted for use of various NFP methods? I would like to see this tool be utilized in future studies on NFP. However, there are other items that I would like to suggest adding to this array. A common characteristic that NFP users indicate that the use of NFP enhances is "self-mastery." I am not sure but I think that self-mastery is still an important value in American life and among the majority of married couples. If this is an important variable in couple relationships, how do various methods of family planning contribute to or detract from this important behavior? Sexual pleasure and intimacy are also important for couple and marital relationships and important characteristics to measure – i.e., as to whether a method of NFP enhances or distracts from intimacy and sexual pleasure. From a holistic perspective spiritual well-being is also important. Does a method of family planning facilitate or detract from a couple's spiritual relationship with God, others and the community. Finally could there be some measure of whether a couple's fertility is integrated or accepted? In other words, if a method of family planning is holistic should it not be accepting and integrating of one's fertility? Would not users of methods of family planning want to know if it enhances dynamics that strengthen marital and family life?

The second exciting aspect of Severy and Jacobs' paper are their reporting for the first time of the overall acceptability, the impact on reproductive knowledge, and the communication across time among couples using the Persona fertility monitor in comparison with couples using condoms. The Persona users could be viewed as a pure NFP group from the sense that they are using a natural method and have not been biased through NFP teaching and by the fact that they were randomly assigned into the group of Persona users.

Severy and Jacobs found that the Persona users (approximately 300 users) in comparison with the (approximately 300) condom users had higher levels of acceptability and reproductive knowledge across 13 cycles of use but that there was essentially no difference in communication. The increase in reproductive knowledge makes sense since condoms use does not inform you about your fertility – they just block it. The acceptability is of interest, in that the use of a fertility monitor (with a red and green light algorithm) is acceptable for use in avoiding pregnancy and that acceptability increased across time. The increase in acceptability is probably due to being more confident in its accuracy in helping to avoid pregnancy. That fact that there was no difference in communication between the two groups is remarkable. Severy and Jacobs speculate it might be due to a "ceiling effect" i.e., the couples already had high levels of communication or that the measure of communication was not sensitive enough. I would speculate the latter.

I would like to see a similar study across time with users of some of the modern methods of NFP and especially in comparison with various family planning methods, such as sterilization, hormonal contraception and barrier methods. And I would like to see further items that measure other positive marital dynamics in the mix of measurement scales.

Severy and Jacobs mentioned at the end of their paper that most people would prefer not to use anything, i.e., any method or technology to avoid or achieve a pregnancy – i.e., to use nothing when dealing with their fertility. I would agree with that assessment. However, if a person ignores or does not at least understand his/her fertility, especially in relation to his/her partner, I wonder how an appreciation of fertility would be attained? NFP couples often have to struggle to integrate their fertility into their relationship but through this struggle they seem to appreciate it more. And couples that have problems with infertility know painfully well how precious the gift of fertility is.

Severy and Jacobs indicated that when couples have to engage their fertility and use something to help them to avoid or achieve pregnancy they prefer a method or technology that is non-invasive, natural, serves as an educational function, provides a positive impact on communication and, of course, that works. I would contend that is what modern NFP is all about. Those are all characteristics of NFP methods as expressed by both teachers and users of NFP. I would also contend that new technology like the Clearplan Easy Fertility Monitor can be an aid for that process. And I agree that there is no "one size fits all" product/method for couples interested in using natural methods. We have a tendency among NFP providers to try to fit one method on all couples and in all circumstances. I believe the message is that we need to tailor the NFP method to the couple and the circumstances.

Finally, to end my short response to Severy's and Jacobs' paper, I would like to quote from Dr. Kyusako Ogino one of the first developers of the Calendar Rhythm Method of family planning and at that time (1932) the chief of the gynecology section of the Takeyama Hospital in Niigata Japan. Dr. Ogino was one of the first persons to think and write about the dynamics of natural methods of family planning. He said that

> Just as the peace between two nations is maintained by mutual good understanding, it is hardly necessary to say that the peace of married couples is created by profound mutual understanding …and understanding that a woman has a fertility and a sterility phase, these alternating periodically. The former period is a holy time, at which the life of new sons and daughters will be created. Thus will the married life be idealized and sanctified (Ogino 1932).

In other words, it is not enough to realize and have the knowledge of the phases of fertility and infertility but also the realization of the holiness of the time for creation. Let us as NFP teachers and researchers continue to strive to understand the dynamics of couple relationships in the use of methods of family planning and let us strive to aid in couples in their peace and understanding. I congratulate professor Larry Severy and Janet Jacobs for their work in contributing to this understanding and hope that he will continue to do so.

Bibliography

Oddens, B.J. 1999. "Women's satisfaction with birth control: a population survey of physical and psychological effects of oral contraceptives, intrauterine devices, condoms, natural family planning, and sterilization among 1466 women." *Contraception* 59:277-286.

Ogino, K. 1934. *Conception Period of Women.* Harrisburg, PA: Medical Arts Publishing.

Correlates of Marital Satisfaction in a Sample of NFP Women

Andrew C. Pollard, Ph.D.(c)
Department of Sociology
State University of New York at Buffalo

Mercedes Arzú-Wilson
President, Family of the Americas Foundation

Abstract

For more than thirty years, NFP researchers have produced a number of studies showing that couples who practice Natural Family Planning are unlike couples who use contraception in important respects, or that the practice of Natural Family Planning contributes to such things as self-esteem, well-being, intimacy, spousal communication and marital satisfaction in ways that contraception does not. Drawing on insights from philosophical personalism, this study evaluates the effect of contraception on women's experience of feeling like an object rather than truly loved by their spouse. Logistic regression analysis finds contraception to have significant positive association with self-reported feeling like an object. Spousal supportiveness and communication are found to be significantly negatively associated with this experience. Spousal communication, heavily promoted through NFP practice, is found to be highly associated with marital satisfaction.

This research was made possible through the assistance and support of the Family of the Americas Foundation

> ... [I]f we start from what utilitarians accept as the basis for the regulation of human behavior we shall never arrive at love. The principle of 'utility' itself, of treating a person as a means to an end, and an end moreover which in this case is pleasure, will always stand in the way of love....
>
> ... But it becomes obvious that if the commandment to love, and the love which is the object of this commandment, are to have any meaning, we must find a basis for them other than the utilitarian premise and the utilitarian system of values. This can only be the personalistic principle and the personalistic norm. This norm, in its negative aspect, states that the person is the kind of good which does not admit of use and cannot be treated as an object of use and as such the means to an end. In its positive form the personalistic norm confirms this: the person is a good towards which the only proper and adequate attitude is love (Wojtyla 1981 [1960], 40-41).

Introduction

For more than thirty years, NFP researchers have produced a number of studies showing that couples who practice Natural Family Planning are unlike couples who use artificial birth control in important respects, or that the practice of Natural Family Planning contributes to such things as self-esteem, well-being, intimacy, spousal communication and marital satisfaction in ways that the use of artificial birth control does not (Marshall and Rowe 1970; McCusker 1977; Tortorici 1979; Borkman and Shivanandan 1984; Klann, Hahlweg and Hank 1988; Boys 1989; Fehring, Lawrence and Sauvage 1989; Fehring and Lawrence 1994). At roughly the same time, philosophical and theological developments, most notably those associated with the work of Karol Wojtyla/Pope John Paul II and the philosophical approach known as *personalism*, have shed new light on the distinction between Natural Family Planning and artificial birth control that NFP researchers take as their object of study (Wojtyla 1981 [1960]; Smith 1991; Schmitz 1993; Smith 1993; Crosby 1996; John Paul II 1997; DeMarco 1999; Shivanandan 1999). Personalism enables us to see how the modalities of acting associated with the practice of Natural Family Planning articulate an axiological orientation fundamentally different from that which is invoked when people use artificial birth control. It thus provides a framework for perceiving the significance of the qualitative and quantitative variations between NFP and contracepting couples that NFP researchers have shown in their empirical investigations. Furthermore, insofar as modalities of acting and the value hierarchies that inform them relate to concrete social structures, the personalist analysis of artificial birth control and Natural Family Planning leads into sociological analysis. In previous work, Pollard (1998) proposed a sociological approach to explaining how Natural Family Planning and artificial birth control express fundamentally different value orientations through their modalities of acting, giving rise to distinct "discourses of fertility." He then showed how these discourses variously reflect or oppose dominant values of modern society.

In the investigation reported in this paper, we test a hypothesis drawn directly from the personalist analysis of artificial birth control. This analysis holds that the use of artificial birth control invokes utilitarian modalities of acting whose effect is to treat the human person, especially the woman, as an object of use. Although this would seem to be an issue of central importance to Natural Family Planning researchers, this study marks the first time a direct test has been conducted on the relationship between contraceptive use and the experience of "feeling like an object." Since personalists emphasize that the opposite of feeling like an object is feeling integrally accepted, known and loved by another as a person, we look for countervailing effects of spousal communication and spousal supportiveness on self-reported "feeling like an object." This provides the basis for a further investigation into the relationship among variables hypothesized to be correlated with marital satisfaction. In particular, we examine the hypothesis, drawn from past research, that the largest contributor to marital satisfaction promoted with regard to NFP practice is couple communication.

Review of Research and Theory

Behavioral research in Natural Family Planning has consistently demonstrated a positive association between the practice of Natural Family Planning, marital satisfaction, and important correlates of marital satisfaction such as couple communication. As early as 1970, Marshall and Rowe found that despite reported difficulties with the Basal Body Temperature Method they practiced, 74% of husbands and 75% of wives in the study believed practicing Natural Family Planning helped their marriages. McCusker (1977) found positive effects of Natural Family Planning on the marital relationship reported in 70.4% of couple responses, with increased communication and deepened love being the most frequently mentioned (1977, 333). Tortorici (1979) found higher levels of self-esteem and marital satisfaction among Catholic married couples who practiced Natural Family Planning compared to those who used artificial birth control and those who had been sterilized. Fehring, Lawrence and Sauvage (1989) added to measures of self-esteem various indices of intimacy and well-being, finding increased levels of both self-esteem and spiritual well-being among couples who practiced Natural Family Planning compared to couples who used artificial birth control.

In 1989 the National Council of Catholic Bishops' Diocesan Development Program for Natural Family Planning commissioned the "Natural Family Planning Nationwide Survey," the first large-scale, multi-center sociological investigation of Natural Family Planning conducted in the United States. Lead researcher Grace A. Boys' analysis of 3,345 questionnaires from practitioner-identified NFP couples in all regions of the U.S. found high reported satisfaction with natural methods, high agreement among NFP spouses in their expression of intimacy, and high agreement that family planning is a mutual responsibility. Similarly, Borkman and Shivanandan (1984), conducted in-depth interviews with NFP couples and found a statistically significant association between the degree to which a couple took joint responsibility for their practice of Natural Family Planning and the degree to which their attitudes toward the abstinence involved in practicing the method were positive and mutually supportive. Content analysis of interviews revealed positive effects of NFP on couples' fertility awareness, sexuality and intimacy, communication, and spiritual well-being. Borkman and Shivanandan also noted that the practice of Natural Family Planning encouraged respect for the woman's body, and that this generalized into what they termed "respect for the personhood of the other, especially the woman" (1984, 62). A later interview study by Fehring and Lawrence (1994) concluded that NFP couples, "felt that their method of family planning helped them to gain a greater fertility awareness, increased communication, provided self-control and confidence, a shared responsibility, enhanced their relationship with God and provided them with more ways of expressing intimacy" (1994, 27).

Klan, Hahlweg and Hank's (1988) study of psychological aspects of NFP practice employed standardized psychological instruments and found that compared to controls, NFP subjects had a generally "positive, uninhibited" attitude toward sexuality, that NFP women felt less "subjectively helpless or dependent on others," and that the marital relationship of NFP couples was marked by a statistically significant decline over time in what the authors termed "the dominant attitude." That is, "The longer NFP is practiced, the more 'considerate, indulgent, forbearing, willing to be tolerant, showing a trusting attitude towards the partner' the participants consider themselves" (1988, 67). Multiple regression analysis showed that the highest percentage of the variance in marital satisfaction was explained by variables directly relevant to the practice of Natural Family Planning. As Klan, Hahlweg and Hank noted of their finding:

> It became apparent that factors concerning the partnership account much more for subjective marital satisfaction and the satisfaction with family life than do factors concerning personality traits or sociodemographic factors. These results lead to the hypothesis that the most important element for the relationship, promoted with regard to NFP practice, is the communication of the partners with one another (1988, 69).

In sum, previous social scientific work on Natural Family Planning has generated an impressive body of evidence showing that Natural Family Planning is positively associated with important correlates of marital satisfaction. These studies pioneered the use of standardized social-psychological instruments with samples of NFP couples and provided valuable templates for survey and interview-based research. Important variables have been identified and methodological sophistication has advanced through the introduction of multivariate methods (Klan, Hahlweg and Hank 1988), calls for statistical control of key variables, such as religiosity (Fehring and Lawrence 1994, 27), and most recently through the articulation of a grounded approach to naturalistic studies with NFP couples (Shinvanandan 1999). A consistent pattern of findings has emerged that provide a warrant for more, and more refined

NFP research going forward. Among the most important of these is the substantial body of evidence linking the practice of Natural Family Planning to enhanced couple communication. There is need to test Klan, Hahlweg and Hank's hypothesis that "the most important element for the relationship, promoted with regard to NFP practice, is the communication of the partners." Such a test should be conducted with statistical control for demographic and other variables, such as religiosity, as called for by Fehring and Lawrence (1994).

At a deeper level, Borkman and Shivanandan's observation of growth in "respect for the personhood of the other, especially the woman" challenges us to place previous research findings of NFP's effects into a broader, personalist perspective. This perspective links *modalities of acting* to *hierarchies of values*. It thus suggests that one explanation for the positive outcomes frequently observed among those who practice Natural Family Planning compared to those who contracept lies in the fact that Natural Family Planning invokes a qualitatively different hierarchy of values in and through the modalities of acting that it deploys. Insofar as Natural Family Planning is constituted of acts such as *recognizing* the signs of fertility produced naturally by the woman's body, *accepting* them as they are, *communicating* their meaning in the context of the spousal relationship, and *abstaining* from sexual intercourse as mutually agreed by the spouses, Natural Family Planning actively engages those who practice it with values centering on acceptance, openness, communication, trust, forbearance, self-control, patience—in short, those values most closely associated with the human expression of *love*. We can thus predict that these modalities of behavior and their associated values which Natural Family Planning promotes will have positive effects on the couple relationship, and will show up empirically as enhanced "well-being" among NFP women and increased communication and marital satisfaction among NFP couples.

By contrast, artificial birth control involves acts in which a chemical substance or technological device is introduced into, typically, the woman's body, in order to alter the natural contingencies of the woman's fertility, usually for the purpose of rendering her sexually available without risk or fear of pregnancy. Personalists assert that artificial birth control, in treating the woman's body and thus the woman herself as an object of chemical or technological alteration, insinuates into the intimate relationship of the spouses modalities of acting that are utilitarian, instrumental, and object-oriented. These modalities bear a particular value orientation centering on efficiency, convenience, autonomy, control, the devaluation of woman in her bodily integrity, and the primacy of pleasure. Thus the intimate union of spouses that is properly meant to be marked by such values as acceptance of the other, trust, mutuality, participation, openness, self-giving and totality becomes colonized by values embedded in the contraceptive modality of acting and in the regime of industrial production and commodity consumption from which it derives. Sociologically, artificial birth control is a "disembedding" mechanism that supplants the woman's natural cycle of fertility by means of a chemical or technological intervention rooted in the abstract-expert system of the biomedical industry (Giddens 1990). It thus insinuates into the spousal relationship a utilitarian modality of acting and a hierarchy of values based upon control (literally, "birth control") while effectively eliminating fertility as an active dimension of the couple relationship and removing it as an experiential domain in which couples might engage in precisely those behaviors and values that are most likely to contribute to feelings of being authentically accepted, known, valued and loved as a person (Figure 1).

Research Hypotheses

Personalist analysis suggests that artificial birth control is associated with a modality of acting and with a constellation of values that are utilitarian and object-oriented. This analysis supplies the first hypothesis tested in this investigation:

Personalist analysis conversely suggests that interpersonal communication and supportive acceptance of the woman typify personalistic relations. This analysis supplies the second hypothesis tested in this investigation:

> *Hypothesis 1*: Use of artificial birth control is significantly associated with an increased likelihood of a woman reporting that she has ever felt like an object rather than truly loved by her spouse

Figure 1. Utilitarian and Personalistic Dimensions of Family Planning as a Function of Interpersonal Communication (Adapted from Shivanandan 1999, 247)

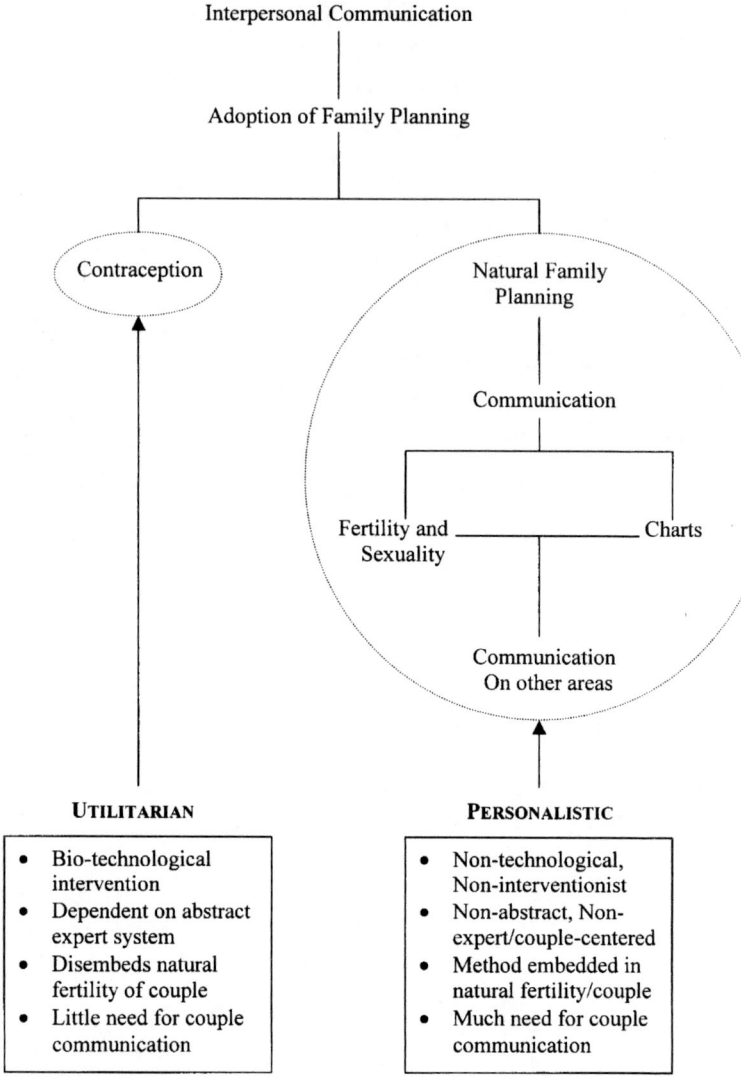

Hypothesis 2: Spousal support for NFP and spousal communication are significantly associated with a decreased likelihood of a woman reporting that she has ever felt like an object rather than truly loved by her spouse.

Personalist analysis and prior NFP research suggest that couple communication is likely to be a major predictor of marital satisfaction. Thus the third hypothesis tested in this investigation is:

Hypothesis 3: Spousal communication strongly predicts marital satisfaction.

Methodology
Data Collection

The data used to examine these hypotheses came from a survey study undertaken during the summer and fall of 2000 by the Family of the Americas Foundation (FAF), an international Natural Family Planning education and promotion organization head-quartered in Dunkirk, Maryland. FAF staff contacted fifteen Family of the Americas NFP teachers in various regions of the U.S. and asked them to solicit former students (women who had taken classes in Natural Family Planning) to participate in the study. Teachers sent names and addresses of willing participants to FAF headquarters. Family of the Americas staff mailed questionnaires to 683 prospective respondents, who were promised $15.00 for completing the questionnaire. 505 women returned completed questionnaires to an independent investigator retained by the Family of the Americas Foundation to provide data entry and descriptive statistical analysis. The survey achieved a 74% response rate.

Characteristics of the Sample

Sampling for the Family of the Americas study was nonrandom, though investigators did attempt to generate a representative sample of women in the U.S. who practice Natural Family Planning. Participants were drawn from 31 U.S. states, making the FAF sample national in scope. To gauge its representativeness, the FAF sample can be compared to the only other national NFP sample, that studied by Grace A. Boys under the auspices of the "Natural Family Planning Nationwide

Survey" (Boys 1989). Ninety two percent of the women in the FAF sample were white, 6% Hispanic and the remaining 2% other. This is comparable to the Boys sample, in which 95% of the women were white. The age of the women in the FAF sample ranged from 21 to 66 years, with a sample mean of 39.8 years (median = 39). This was considerably older than the mean age of 31.7 years for women in the Boys sample. On average, women in the FAF sample were married longer (15.4 years) than women in the Boys sample (8.6 years).

Measures of education in the two samples are not directly comparable, although in general, women in the FAF sample were highly educated: 45% were college graduates and 15% reported completing a Master's degree or higher. Boys reported the "average level of education" for the women in her study as 2.7 years of college. Ninety one percent of women in the FAF sample were Roman Catholic, compared to 83.2% in the Boys sample. Another 8% in the FAF sample described themselves as Protestant/Christian and only four respondents out of the total sample of 505 specifically indicated no religion. Religious attendance was high among the women in the FAF sample, with 58% of respondents describing themselves as weekly attendees and 30% describing themselves as attending church more than once a week. This appears roughly comparable to the Boys sample, which showed "average" church attendance as being about once a week.

Median income in the FAF sample fell between $50,000 and $60,000 annually, which is higher but still comparable after adjusting for inflation to the $35,000 to $40,000 median range reported by Boys. Approximately 20% of the respondents in the FAF sample described themselves as working full-time, with an additional 26% describing themselves as part-time workers. Forty two percent of the FAF sample described their occupation as that of a homemaker. This is very close to the 39% of women in the Boys sample who described themselves as homemakers. Ninety eight percent of women the FAF sample identified themselves as currently married. Only one woman described herself as currently divorced, though 18 women (roughly 4%) described themselves as having been divorced at some time during their life. There were no statistics on divorce provided in the Boys study.

Use of Artificial Birth Control among Women in the FAF Sample

Since the effects of artificial birth control are a centerpiece of this investigation it is worthwhile looking in some detail at the pattern of its use reported in the FAF data. Although these data come from a sample of women known to have learned and practiced Natural Family Planning, 329 women in the sample (65%) reported having used artificial birth control. On average, these women reported having used 2 contraceptive methods during their lives, and 24% reported having used three or more contraceptive methods. The remaining 35% of the women in the FAF sample indicated that they had never used a contraceptive and had only ever practiced Natural Family Planning. One hundred thirty four women in the FAF sample of 505 (26.5%) indicated that they were not currently practicing Natural Family Planning, and 49 women (9.7%) reported that they were currently using some form of artificial birth control. However, nearly half of these 49 women reported that they were *also* currently practicing Natural Family Planning, suggesting that they may have been practicing some form of a "combination method."

The cohort of 49 women who reported currently using some form of artificial birth control represents a subgroup of the sample of NFP women who, for one reason or another (data were not available), decided either to discontinue their practice of Natural Family Planning or to modify it by means of adding a contraceptive. This cohort was not statistically different from the rest of the sample in terms of age, education or income. However, the mean religious attendance of this cohort (7.18) was significantly lower than the rest of the sample (8.13), $t\,(df/50.879)$[1] $= -3.379$, $p=.001$, although it was still relatively high (nearly every week). It is not possible to ascertain from the data whether lower religious attendance was a stable characteristic of this cohort that preceded their choice to use artificial birth control, or whether their choice to adopt artificial birth control subsequently affected their religious observance. It is interesting to note, however, that while the cohort showed significantly lower religious attendance than the main sample, there was no statistically significant difference between the cohort and the rest of the sample with respect to the question, "How important is religion in your life?"

The cohort reporting current use of artificial birth control had a slightly higher mean number of sex partners over the life course (2.47) compared to the main sample (1.89), t (df/53.786) = 2.025, p=.048. A 2 x 2 contingency table analysis also showed that membership in the artificial birth control-using cohort was significantly related with premarital sexual involvement c^2 (df/1, n=491) = 7.265, p=.007. However, there was no statistically significant relationship between membership in the cohort and self-reported ever having felt like an object rather than truly loved by one's spouse, and there was no significant difference in the frequency of spousal communication between the cohort reporting current use of a contraceptive and the rest of the sample.

Satisfaction with spousal communication was significantly lower in the cohort indicating current use of artificial birth control (5.82) compared to the main sample (6.50), t (df/55.402) = -2.583, p=.012. Similarly, the cohort reported significantly higher mean difficulty with abstinence (4.34) than the rest of the sample (3.66), t (df/32.187) = 2.613, p=.014, significantly lower spousal supportiveness during abstinence (4.56) compared to the sample (5.33), t (df/28.436) = -3.008, p=.005, and significantly lower spousal supportiveness for the practice of NFP overall (5.10) than the rest of the sample (5.64), t (df/30.628) = -2.721, p=.011. A reasonable interpretation of these findings is that difficulty practicing Natural Family Planning and/or a lack of spousal support and communication may have led these women to opt for artificial birth control, either instead of the practice of Natural Family Planning or in addition to it. There was no statistically significant difference in mean frequency of intercourse between the cohort reporting current use of artificial birth control and the rest of the sample, and women in the cohort were no more likely than the rest of the sample to have been divorced.

The 109 women in the sample who reported currently practicing neither Natural Family Planning nor artificial birth control ranged in age from 27 to 66 years and comprised two likely subsets of women: younger women who were open to achieving a pregnancy and older women who were beyond childbearing age. The mean age of this non-NFP/non-contraceptive-using cohort (46.45) is significantly older than the rest of the sample (37.81), t (df/134.042) = 8.055, p=.000, suggesting support for the interpretation that the cohort included women no longer practicing Natural Family Planning due to their age.

Dependent Variables

Two dependent variables were used in this investigation. The question, "Have you ever felt like an object rather than truly loved by your husband, fiancé, or boyfriend?" was used to test hypothesis 1. Response categories provided for this question were yes/no, yielding a dichotomous coding (0 for no, 1 for yes) suitable for use in a logistic regression analysis. The dependent variable used to test hypothesis 2 was the question, "If you are currently married or in a relationship,

Table 1. Dependent Variables from FAF Survey with Valid N, Missing Values, Means and Standard Deviations				
Variable	Valid N	Missing	Mean	S.D.
nfp1_25. Have you ever felt like an object rather than truly loved by your husband, fiancé, or boyfriend? 1=Yes, 0=No	488	17	.3607	.4807
p2_1. If you are currently married or in a relationship, taking all things into consideration, how would describe your marriage or relationship? 4=Very happy, 3=Pretty happy, 2=Not too happy, 1=Don't know.	497	8	3.55	.6367

taking all things into consideration, how would describe your marriage or relationship?" Response categories included: very happy, pretty happy, not too happy, and don't know. This item was reverse-coded so that higher scores reflected greater happiness in marriage.

Independent Variables

Three independent variables were studied in this investigation. The first was contraceptive use. This was measured by means of a variable created from totaling the number of different contraceptive methods each respondent identified ever having used in her lifetime. The computed contraceptive use variable ranged from 0 to 5 contraceptive

Table 2. Independent Variables from FAF Survey with Valid N, Missing Values, Means and Standard Deviations

Variable	Valid N	Missing	Mean	S.D.
Contraceptive use (Range=0-5)	505	0	1.4317	1.3481
Spousal Support for NFP (Range=1-6)	393	112	5.3868	0.9492
Spousal Communication (Range=1-7)	498	7	5.2038	1.2508

methods ever used. From this, a second, dichotomous contraceptive use variable was created for use in the investigation's initial contingency table analysis. This variable indicated simply if a respondent had ever used a contraceptive (coded 1) or not (coded 0).

The second independent variable of interest was spousal support for NFP. This was an index variable computed from two separate survey items: "During abstinence from sexual intercourse, how supportive is your husband, fiancé or boyfriend?" and " In general, how supportive is your husband, fiancé, or boyfriend in your practice of Natural Family Planning?" In the survey, these items were worded in such a way that only women who were currently practicing Natural Family Planning were invited to respond. Thus the numbers of responses for these items were considerably lower relative to the sample N of 505. Response categories for these questions included: very supportive, supportive, somewhat supportive, somewhat unsupportive, unsupportive, very unsupportive. Items were reverse-coded prior to computation of the index so as to render a higher number indicative of higher support for NFP. Reliability analysis yielded a Cronbach's Alpha of .7925 for the index.

The second independent variable of interest in the study was spousal communication. This was also an index variable that was computed from two separate survey items: "How frequently do you have intimate conversations with your husband, fiancé, or boyfriend?" and "How satisfied are you with your communication with you husband, fiancé, or boyfriend?" Response categories for frequency of intimate conversations included: none, once or twice, about once a month, 2 or 3 times a month, about once a week, 2 or 3 times a week, 4 or more times a week. Response categories for satisfaction with communication included: extremely satisfied, very satisfied, satisfied, somewhat satisfied, somewhat dissatisfied, dissatisfied, very dissatisfied, extremely dissatisfied. These items were reverse-coded prior to computation of the index so as to render a higher number indicative of higher satisfaction with communication. Reliability analysis yielded a Cronbach's Alpha of .7731 for the index. (Table 3 begins below and continues on next page.)

Control Variables

Education, income and religious attendance were the chief control variables in the investigation. Since the experience of ever having felt like an object rather than truly loved could be related to one's sexual history or current pattern of sexual activity, the number of past sexual partners the woman reported having and the woman's reported frequency of sexual intercourse were included as controls.

Procedure

A two-by-two contingency table analysis was conducted to test for a basic relationship between contraceptive use and the experience of ever having felt like an object rather than truly loved by one's spouse (hypothesis 1). Following this, a logistic regression analysis was

Table 3. Control Variables from FAF Survey with Valid N, Missing Values, Means & Standard Deviations

Variable	Valid N	Missing	Mean	S.D.
p3_4. What was the highest grade or year of schooling you completed? 1=Some high school or less, 2=Finished high school or equivalent, 3=Vocational, trade, business school, 4=Some college or 2-year degree, 5=Finished college, 4 to 5 year degree, 6=Master's degree or equivalent, other advanced degree	499	6	4.4770	1.1741

p3_13. About how much total income, before taxes, did your family make in 1999? 1=$4,999 or less, 2=$5,000 to $7,999, 3=$8,000 to $12,499, 4=$12,500 to $14,999, 5=$15,000 to $17,499, 6=$17,500 to $19,999, 7=$20,000 to $22,499, 8=$22,500 to $24,999, 9=$25,000 to $29,999, 10=$30,000 to $34,999, 11=$35,000 to $39,999, 12=$40,000 to $49,999, 13=$50,000 to $59,999, 14=$60,000 to $74,999, 15=$75,000 or over.	472	33		2.4?
p3_11. How often do you attend religious services? 1=Never, 2=Less than once a year, 3=About once or twice a year, 4=Several times a year, 5=About once a month, 6=2 to 3 times a month, 7=Nearly every week, 8=Every week, 9=Several times a week	502	3	8.0339	1.1$
nfp1_26. Thinking back over your lifetime, how many men have you had sexual relations with, even if only one time? 1=One, 2=Two, 3=Three, 4=Four, 5=Five, 6=Six or more	481	24	1.9543	1.6$
nfp1_22. About how often did you have sex in the last 12 months? 1=None, 2=Once or twice, 3=About once a month, 4=2 or 3 times a month, 5=About once a week, 6=2 or 3 times a week, 7=4 or more times a week.	488	17	4.7111	1.18

employed to model the effects of various control and independent variables on the likelihood that a woman reported having felt like an object (hypotheses 1 & 2). To assess the basic pattern and strength of the associations among variables hypothesized to be related to marital satisfaction, zero-order correlation coefficients were computed and tabulated. Afterwards, a multiple regression analysis was performed in order to ascertain the relative percentage of the variance in marital satisfaction explained by couple communication, controlling for demographic variables, sexual history, reported feeling like an object and spousal support for NFP (hypothesis 3).

Results

Table 4 summarizes results of a crosstabulation showing the basic structure of the association between contraceptive use and feeling like an object among women in the FAF sample. Missing data reduced the cases in analysis from 505 to 488. The basic form of the association was as predicted in hypothesis 1. Seventy-four percent of women who never used a contraceptive also reported never having felt like an object rather than loved by their spouse. This is a significantly higher rate of never having felt like an object compared to the 59% of women who reported using artificial birth control at some time in their lives. Likewise, 40% of women who used a contraceptive compared to 26% who did not reported feeling like an object rather than loved by their spouse. In support of hypothesis 1, a chi-square test indicates that contraceptive use was significantly associated with ever having felt like an object rather than truly loved, c^2 (df/1, n=488) = 10.399, $p=.001$.

The association between contraceptive use and self-reported feeling like an object is expanded below by means of a logistic regression analysis. This analytic technique is for use with a dichotomous (0,1) dependent variable. In logistic regression analysis, the logged odds of the dependent variable occurring are computed as a function of its linear relationship to an independent variable or variables. Five models were included in the logistic analysis summarized in table 5. In model one, the control variables for education, income, and religiosity were included in the equation. To these were added in model 2 the control variables for sexual history and frequency of intercourse. In models 3 through 5, the three independent variables of interest

Table 4. Crosstabulation of Ever Felt Like an Object with Ever Used Artificial birth control

	Ever Used Artificial birth control?				Total	
	No		Yes			
Ever Felt Like an object? *No*	74%	123	59%	189	312	
Yes	26%	44	41%	132	176	
Total	100%	167	100%	321	488	

χ^2 (df/1, n=488) = 10.399, $p=.001$.

were added: contraceptive use, spousal support for NFP and spousal communication.

Logistic estimates (Table 5) were computed to determine the relative importance of sociodemographic, sexual history, contraceptive use, NFP support, and communication variables on the logged odds of a woman reporting ever having felt like an object rather that truly loved by her spouse. As previously discussed, the index of spousal support for NFP included items that invited only women who were currently practicing NFP to respond. Inclusion of this index and missing values reduced the cases in the analysis from 505 to 333. Based on the coefficient to its standard error, three variables were consistently significant predictors of a woman reporting having felt like an object: contraceptive use, spousal support for NFP and spousal communication. Testing of model 5 coefficients utilizing a Bayesian Information Criterion (BIC) procedure (Pampel 2000, 31) showed spousal communication to be a very strongly significant predictor of the dependent variable, followed by contraceptive use (less strong) and spousal support for NFP use, (weak but still significant).

Exponentiating the coefficient, subtracting one and multiplying by 100 shows the percentage change in the odds of feeling like an object rather than truly loved by one's spouse for a one-unit change in each predictor (Pampel 2000, 36). In model 5, for each contraceptive method a woman reported using (beginning with 0), her odds of ever having felt like an object rather than truly loved by her spouse increased by $(.336e-1)100$, or 40%, controlling for sociodemographic factors, sexual history, spousal support for NFP, and spousal communication. This finding provides support for hypothesis 1. A one-unit increase in spousal support for Natural Family Planning reduced the odds of a woman reporting that she has ever felt like an object by $(-.423e-1)100$ or 34.5%, controlling for all other variables in the equation. A one-unit increase in spousal communication reduced the odds of a woman ever having felt like an object by $(-.594e-1)100$ or 44.8%, controlling for sociodemographic, sexual history, spousal support for NFP, and contraceptive use. These findings provide support for hypothesis 2.

The chi-square value of the test of model 5 coefficients (70.917) showed a significant improvement in prediction of the dependent variable with the inclusion of the modeled independent variables, as

Table 5. Logistic Estimates of Reported Ever Felt Like an Object Rather Than Truly Loved by Spouse

Variables	Model 1	Model 2	Model 3	Model 4	Model 5
Education	-.062 (.102)	-.079 (.103)	-.090 (.109)	-.127 (.113)	-.099 (.115)
Income	-.076 (.049)	-.082 (.050)	-.069 (.053)	-.059 (.055)	-.087 (.057)
Religious Attendance	.017 (.105)	.055 (.107)	.093 (.116)	.083 (.117)	.122 (.122)
Number of Sexual Partners		-.137* (.069)	.136 (.072)	.131 (.076)	.033 (.083)
Frequency of Intercourse		-.086 (.108)	.026 (.118)	.218 (.130)	.193 (.132)
Contraceptive Use			.360** (.096)	.311** (.101)	.336** (.104)
Spousal Support for NFP				-.724** (.152)	-.423** (.162)
Spousal Communication					-.594** (.139)
Constant	.568 (1.08)	.536 (1.22)	.168 (1.25)	3.187 (1.49)	3.901 (1.53)
-2 Log Likelihood Initial	437.558				
Model	433.844	429.093	414.609	386.115	366.640
χ^2	3.714	8.465	22.948**	51.443**	70.917**

*$p \leq .05$ **$p \leq .01$ Standard errors are in parentheses.

compared to the baseline (initial) model. Utilizing the method of correlating the predicted probabilities generated by the model with the dependent variable as a measure of the goodness of the fit of the model to the data (Pampel 2000, 50), yields a pseudo-R^2 value for model 5 of .205 (R = .453). The pseudo-R^2 is roughly analogous to the percentage of variance explained (R^2) in an OLS regression model. Model 5 improved prediction of the dependent variable by slightly over 20%. Contraceptive use significantly increased the likelihood that a woman in the FAF sample ever felt like an object rather than truly loved by her spouse (hypothesis 1), and spousal communication and support for NFP significantly decreased that likelihood (hypothesis 2).

Table 6 (see facing page) displays zero-order correlation coefficients for the four main variables considered so far—contraceptive use, feeling like an object, spousal support for NFP and spousal communication. The table also shows the correlations of these variables with marital satisfaction. The direction of all coefficients was as expected. Contraceptive use was positively associated with feeling like an object, and was negatively associated with spousal support, communication and marital satisfaction, though with diminishing statistical significance. Feeling like an object was significantly negatively associated with spousal support, spousal communication and marital satisfaction. Marital satisfaction was significantly associated with spousal support for NFP, and marital satisfaction was also significantly associated with spousal communication. Spousal communication had the strongest association to marital satisfaction of all the variables analyzed (.651). This finding provides initial support for hypothesis 3.

The preceding analysis of correlation coefficients was expanded by means of a multiple regression analysis investigating the effects of several control and independent variables on marital satisfaction. As before, five models were included in the regression analysis. Model 1 included only the control variables for education, income, and religiosity. Model 2 added variables for sexual history and frequency of intercourse. In models 3 through 5, the three independent variables of interest were added: felt like an object, spousal support for NFP and spousal communication. Of particular interest in this analysis was assessing the impact of spousal communication on marital satisfaction.

Table 6. Zero-Order Correlation Coefficients For Contraceptive Use, Felt Like an Object, NFP Support, Spousal Communication and Marital Satisfaction

Variables	1	2	3	4	5
1 Contraceptive Use	1.000				
2 Ever Felt Like an Object	.217**	1.000			
3 Spousal Support for NFP	-.140**	-.304**	1.000		
4 Spousal Communication	-.094*	-.333**	.475**	1.000	
5 Marital Satisfaction	-.014	-.346**	.398**	.651**	1.000

*$p \leq .05$ **$p \leq .01$

Regression coefficients (Table 7: see next page) were computed to determine the relative effects of sociodemographic, sexual history, felt like an object, NFP support, and communication variables on marital satisfaction. Inclusion of the index of spousal support for NFP and missing values reduced the cases in the analysis from 505 to 332. Based on the coefficient to its standard error, income was the only demographic control variable that had a consistent, significant (though small) effect on marital satisfaction. Frequency of sexual intercourse had a significant effect in Model 2, but then dropped to insignificance in subsequent models. Overall, having felt like an object rather than truly loved by one's spouse significantly reduced a woman's reported marital satisfaction in all models that included this variable. However, this effect weakened substantially with the addition of spousal supportiveness and spousal communication to the regression equation. The addition of each of these variables increased explanation of marital satisfaction. Controlling for demographic, sexual history and feeling like an object variables, NFP supportiveness explained over 10% of the variance in marital satisfaction, and spousal communication explained an additional 17%, even after controlling for spousal support for NFP. Of the over 45% of the variance in marital satisfaction explained in the full model (5), the largest proportion explained by a single variable was contributed by couple communication. This finding provides support for hypothesis 3, that couple communication explains a substantial proportion of marital satisfaction.

Discussion

Previous research (Klann, Hahlweg & Hank 1988) suggested that the most important element for the spousal relationship promoted with

Table 7. OLS Regression Coefficients of Marital Satisfaction

Variables	Model 1	Model 2	Model 3	Model 4	Model 5
Education	-.029 (.030)	-.027 (.029)	-.035 (.028)	-.031 (.026)	-.031 (.023)
Income	.047** (.015)	.048** (.014)	.041** (.014)	.037** (.013)	.035** (.011)
Religious Attendance	-.028 (.030)	-.039 (.030)	-.035 (.028)	-.045 (.027)	-.042 (.023)
Number of Sexual Partners		-.038 (.020)	-.025 (.019)	-.025 (.018)	-.020 (.016)
Frequency of Intercourse		.120** (.030)	.112 (.029)	.081 (.028)	-.013 (.026)
Ever Felt Like an Object			-.398** (.065)	-.261** (.064)	-.128* (.064)
Spousal Support for NFP				.219** (.032)	.083** (.031)
Spousal Communication					.276** (.028)
Constant	3.345 (.313)	2.909 (.345)	3.154 (.330)	2.184 (.340)	1.783 (.340)
R^2	.031	.087	.182	.284	.453
$R^2 \Delta$	.031	.056	.095	.102	.169
$F \Delta$	3.519*	9.947**	37.864**	46.022**	100.105**

*$p \leq .05$, **$p \leq .01$. Standard errors are in parentheses.

regard to NFP is the communication of the spouses with one another. This investigation provides support for that hypothesis. While this investigation did not inquire into whether the practice of Natural Family Planning *contributes* to spousal communication, it did find that spousal communication is highly correlated (.651) with marital satisfaction, and after controlling for education, income, religiosity, sexual history, feeling like an object and NFP supportiveness, spousal communication explains a substantial proportion (nearly 17%) of the variance in marital satisfaction in the FAF sample. Overall, spousal support for NFP and spousal communication were strong correlates of marital satisfaction, a finding both in line with previous NFP research and supportive of the personalist analysis of Natural Family Planning. This analysis suggests that Natural Family Planning engages spouses in a modality of acting that encourages interpersonal communication and mutual supportiveness through the joint management of fertility that the method facilitates. It also illuminates how NFP is embedded in a hierarchy of values centered on the integral acceptance of the human person, particularly the woman. Thus, insofar as the practice of Natural Family Planning promotes couple communication and supportiveness, as well as valuing the woman in her bodily integrity above sexual pleasure, personalism predicts the method is likely to enhance the marital satisfaction of the couple.

The investigation found that use of artificial birth control increased the odds of a woman feeling like an object rather than truly loved by her spouse in the FAF sample. This was true even after controlling for demographic, sexual history, spousal support for NFP and spousal communication variables. Spousal support for NFP and spousal communication significantly decreased the odds of a woman feeling like an object rather than truly loved by her spouse. The largest single effect in all logistic models evaluated was provided by couple communication, which substantially reduced the odds of a woman reporting that she has ever felt like an object rather than truly loved by her spouse. Based upon this analysis, it is reasonable to conclude that insofar as the practice of Natural Family Planning contributes to couple communication and personalist values, it also decreases the likelihood that a woman will feel like an object rather than loved by her spouse.

Another dimension of these findings goes more deeply to the personalist analysis of artificial birth control and to its related sociological analysis. The findings of this investigation suggest that artificial birth control has its own effect on whether a woman will report feeling like an object, above and beyond any effect mediated solely by couple communication. That is, even after controlling for couple communication and spousal support, artificial birth control was still significantly associated with women feeling like an object rather than truly loved. It thus appears to be the case that artificial birth control cannot be used without engendering a "utilitarian" effect in some women, even where couple communication might be good. Use of artificial birth control itself appears to be significantly associated with some women reporting feeling like an object rather than truly loved. This comports with the personalist analysis of artificial birth control, but it also points to the sociological analysis of artificial birth control as a disembedding, technical-instrumental intervention that insinuates utilitarian values directly into the intimate relations of spouses.

A central assumption among many who use and promote artificial birth control is that artificial birth control is technologically "neutral." That is, the contraceptive itself bears no intrinsic value orientation that might impact those who use it. The contraceptive simply renders a woman able to "control" her fertility, and thus, the argument goes, the range of artificial birth control's effects is limited to where, when and how it is used by individuals. The materialist and utilitarian philosophical anthropology underlying such an analysis stresses the autonomy of the individual and brooks no analysis of the human person as a *relation* who is infused with value-meanings that have significant effects. Thus promoters of artificial birth control assert that there is nothing about the contraceptive itself that is capable of producing a feeling of "objectness" in women. If a woman does report such a feeling, the reason lies not with the contraceptive—which is simply a "product"—but rather with the woman herself and with the nature of the sexual relationship in which she finds herself.

Such an analysis, however, fails to recognize that many technological innovations are not at all "neutral" in their effects on human persons. Moreover, it utterly fails to recognize the uniqueness of the contraceptive product, which is a device or drug whose singular purpose is precisely to alter the natural contingencies of a woman's body, and therefore the woman *herself*. It is ironic that feminist supporters of artificial birth control, who in other arenas of argument typically assert the "integrality" of women's experience—usually including the integrality of a woman's body with her whole person—demur from such an assertion when the issue is artificial birth control. Women should be viewed in their totality in all other arenas of social life, yet when it comes to artificial birth control advocates argue that a woman can chemically or technologically alter herself with *no* consequence to her personhood. Personalism, with its more adequate anthropology centering on the relational and valuational aspects of human personhood, refutes such an assertion and suffers no such inconsistency of argument. It links modalities of acting toward human persons with the discrete hierarchies of values that inform such modalities. It thus predicts that artificial birth control *can* and frequently *does* convey a feeling of objectness to women who use it precisely because it is a modality of acting that arises from within a utilitarian constellation of values and takes as its sole aim the insinuation of those values into the relationship of a woman with her own body and with her spouse.

Sociosemiotically, the artificial birth control is not neutral. It is an industrial product that is encoded with values derived from a system of industrial control and manipulation. It is a disembedding mechanism that supplants the natural cycle of fertility with a regime of control achieved through the application of a technical-instrumental intervention. While it can be argued that modern people use many industrial products without consequence to their personhood, it must be borne in mind that artificial birth control is a *unique* industrial product. Its sole function is to change fundamentally the contingencies of a woman's body with respect to one of its most intimate, relational functions. Insofar as artificial birth control is a social practice, it necessarily articulates the values embedded in the social structures and processes from which it derives. Sociologists have long studied such phenomena. Personalist analysis simply helps put artificial birth control on the sociological radar screen by drawing attention to *why* there might be an association between using artificial birth control and feeling like an object rather than truly loved as a person.

It can be objected that the women in the FAF sample who used artificial birth control were not representative of all women who use artificial birth control. They came to the attention of researchers through their practice of Natural Family Planning, and NFP may have been chosen by these women in the light of their previous experience with artificial birth control. Thus the contraceptively experienced women in the FAF sample could be biased in their view of artificial birth control in a way that makes them fundamentally different from other women who use artificial birth control. "Feeling like an object" may have been an awareness that came through the practice of Natural Family Planning; it may not be endemic to the use of artificial birth control at all. Respondents in the FAF sample may have drawn a comparison between artificial birth control and NFP and then answered the survey in the way they thought fit the objectives of the researcher. Although there is little in the survey data to suggest such an effect and the questions about use of artificial birth control and feeling like an object were structurally separate in the questionnaire, a replication of the current investigation would want to employ independent samples of NFP women and non-NFP contracepting women.

Conclusion

The personalist analysis of artificial birth control predicts that its use is likely to insinuate utilitarian values and modalities of acting into the relationship of spouses. In contrast, personalism provides a framework for understanding the benefits of Natural Family Planning that previous behavioral NFP research has demonstrated. Natural Family Planning engages couples in a modality of acting centered on recognizing, accepting, communicating, and abiding with a woman's body in its integrity. In so doing, NFP engages couples in a hierarchy of values centered on *love* and fundamentally opposed to *use*. Correlates of marital satisfaction frequently seen in NFP women may be explained by the fact that Natural Family Planning is an intensely personalistic practice. There is thus need to integrate insights from personalism into social scientific research with NFP couples. This study has attempted to be a first step in that direction.

Bibliography

Borkman, T. 1979. "A Social-Science Perspective of Research Issues for Natural Family Planning." *International Review of Natural Family Planning* 3(4):331-354.

Borkman, T. and Shivanandan, M. 1984. "The Impact of Natural Family Planning on Selected Aspects of the Couple Relationship." *International Review of Natural Family Planning* 8(4):58-66.

Boys, G.A. 1989. *Natural Family Planning Nationwide Survey: Final Report to the National Conference of Catholic Bishops.* Irvington, NJ: Diocesan Development Program for Natural Family Planning.

Crosby, J.F. 1996. *The Selfhood of the Human Person.* Washington, DC: Catholic University of America Press.

DeMarco, D. 1999. *New Perspectives on Contraception.* Dayton, OH: One More Soul.

Fehring, R., and Lawrence, D.M.. 1994. "Spiritual Well-being, Self-esteem and Intimacy Among Couples Using Natural Family Planning." *Linacre Quarterly* 6(3):18-29.

Fehring, R., Lawrence, D.M., and Sauvage, C.M. 1989. "Self-esteem, Spiritual Well-being, and Intimacy: A Comparison Among Couples Using NFP." *International Review of Natural Family Planning* 13(3-4):227-236.

Giddens, A.1990. *The Consequences of Modernity.* Stanford, CA: Stanford University Press.

John Paul II. 1997. *The Theology of the Body: Human Love in the Divine Plan.* Boston, MA: Pauline Books & Media.

Klann, N., Hahlweg, K., and Hank, G. 1988. "Psychological Aspects of NFP Practice." *International Journal of Fertility* (Supplement):65-69.

Marshall, J. and Rowe, B.1970. "Psychologic Aspects of the Basal Body Temperature Method of Regulating Births." *Fertility and Sterility* 21(1): 14-19.

McCusker, M.P. 1977. "NFP and the Marital Relationship: The Catholic University of America Study." *International Review of Natural Family Planning* 1(4):331-340.

Pollard, A. 1999. *Discourse of Fertility: Towards a Sociosemiotic Conceptualization of Natural Family Planning.* Poster Presentation at the Eighteenth Annual Meeting of the American Association of Natural Family Planning, Lowell, MA, July 23, 1999.

Schmitz, K.L. 1993. *At the Center of the Human Drama: The Philosophical Anthropology of Karol Wojtyla/Pope John Paul II.* Washington, DC: Catholic University of America Press.

Shivanandan, M.1999. *Crossing the Threshold of Love: A New Vision of Marriage.* Washington, DC: Catholic University of America Press.

Smith, J. 1991. *Humanae Vitae a Generation Later.* Washington, DC: Catholic University of America Press.

Smith, J., ed. 1993. *Why Humanae Vitae Was Right: A Reader.* San Francisco: Ignatius.

Tortorici, J. 1979. "Conception Regulation, Self-esteem, and Marital Satisfaction Among Catholic Couples." *International Review of Natural Family Planning* 3:191-205.

Wojtyla, K. (Pope John Paul II). 1981 [1960]. *Love and Responsibility.* San Francisco: Ignatius.

Note

[1] t-tests reported in this section reflect conservative estimates (equal variances not assumed), as determined by Levene's test of equality of variances. All p-values reported are two-tailed tests.

Response to Pollard and Arzú-Wilson: Correlates of Marital Satisfaction in a Sample of NFP Women

Julie Krause, B.S.N., R.N.
Diocesan NFP Coordinator, Diocese of Madison, Wisconsin

General Comments

Pollard's study looks at "something old" and "something new." The "something old" is marital satisfaction as it relates to communication. The "something new" is addressing whether NFP trained women, who used contraception in the past, report the experience of feeling "like an object" rather than feeling "loved" by their husbands. This is an interesting question in light of the NFP Community's ongoing attempts to demonstrate that contraception is harmful to women and couples, and that NFP is beneficial.

The theoretical underpinnings of the study are thoroughly constructed and have been discussed and studied previously by other researchers. The hypotheses follow directly from the theory.

Study Strengths

A major strength of this study is the large number (505) of subjects taken from across the U.S. Several comparisons to similar national surveys were made to determine the representative value of the sample. In most categories, demographics compared favorably with the other surveys.

The author notes that NFP trained couples who use contraception are possibly not representative of the general population of contraception users. Thus, the results may not generalize to non-NFP trained women.

Although there is no control group in this study, Pollard attempts to control for demographic factors, religious attendance and relationship factors (i.e., spousal support and communication) when evaluating the question of NFP use and "feeling like an object." Other studies have documented the relationship between religious practice, family income, communication and high levels of marital satisfaction.

Study weaknesses

Any study of human behavior is likely to have weak points. I found three areas where I felt the study could have been stronger.

First, the question, "Have you ever felt like an object, rather than truly loved by your husband?" is somewhat vague and can be interpreted in several ways. There is no demonstration of reliability or validity of this question. Since this is a first study using this measure, I would have expected the author to discuss the issue of reliability. As a reader, I assume the survey used only this single item, thus there are no related questions in the survey that would help to establish reliability. A follow up survey that included several questions relating to "feeling like an object" would create a more reliable measurement.

In the analysis section of the paper, multiple models were presented to evaluate the correlation of "feeling like an object" with the independent variables. I found this confusing and unnecessary. Moving directly to model five would have been simpler, without compromising the findings. In addition to being confusing, the larger number of statistical analyses increases the likelihood of spurious (false positive) results.

The regression analysis regarding Marital Satisfaction did not include "Contraceptive Use" as a predictor variable. This is a curious omission in a study where the theory so strongly states that contraceptive use will undermine couple communication.

As a correlational study, the results are significant and support the hypotheses. In the discussion, causation is implied, or in some cases stated directly, (p. 24) and causality has not been demonstrated in this study. This is perhaps the most problematic piece of the report.

The Abstract and the Results sections of the paper clearly state the findings. However, the detailed presentation of "personalist theory" in the Discussion section blurs the distinction between what is demonstrated by research and what remains theoretical. The theory "predicts that contraception can and does convey a feeling of objectiveness to women who use it…" Such a broad theoretical prediction of causal relationship has not been demonstrated by this data. While it is appropriate to relate the theory to the study findings, Pollard does so in such a way that it would be easy to assume that this study's findings support the theory, when it does not. The detailed theoretical discussion would be more appropriate for a "Review of Research and Theory." Here in the Discussion section, it bogs down the findings, and leads to confusion.

Finally, this study demonstrates a correlation between contraceptive use and "feeling like an object," which can be generalized only to women trained in NFP. Pollard notes that learning NFP may alter a woman's perception of contraception in ways that make women knowledgeable in NFP fundamentally different from other women. While he acknowledges this is a weakness of the study, (p. 27) in other places he writes as if this weakness did not exist, and that the correlation found in this study is applicable to the general population. (p. 26)

Conclusion

I encourage those in the NFP Community to use and share this study, but to do so within the confines of the study findings. To do otherwise undermines the credibility of NFP research of all types and contributes to the perception that NFP is not "scientific enough" for acceptance by the community at large, especially the medical community.

Pollard's study is a good first step in the process of validating the "personalist theory." More studies need to be done, especially if the NFP Community wishes to support the theory that NFP increases couple communication. To date we have anecdotal studies, and correlational studies, but no studies that demonstrate causal relationships. Here is the new frontier for NFP research, and I look forward to seeing more work from Andrew Pollard.

Preliminary Comparison of Algorithm-Interpreted Fertility Monitor Readings with Established Natural Family Planning Methods

Jennine Regas, M.S.
Philip Regas, M.B.A.
Zetek, Inc Aurora, Colorado

Abstract

Women experienced in established NFP methods provided records of 53 cycles. Twenty-four cycles were contributed by women in the 2001 study. An additional 29 cycles from an earlier study were evaluated retrospectively using the OvaCue® algorithm. In addition to maintaining their ongoing fertility observations, all subjects took oral electrolyte readings daily, vaginal electrolyte readings during the fertile window as specified by the algorithm, and urinary luteinizing hormone (uLH) tests on days identified by the algorithm as days of maximum fertility. The fertile window (FW) was defined as the five days preceding ovulation and the day of ovulation (Wilcox, et al.1995). Each method was examined to determine how closely it defined the FW both as a means to achieve and to avoid conception. The OvaCue and the Sympto-Thermal methods were closely correlated, especially in defining the end of the FW. The OvaCue was found to be more effective than other methods in determining the beginning of the FW. Overall, the OvaCue algorithm analysis correctly identified all FW days in over 99% of cycles. Sympto-Thermal Method identified 87.38% of FW days. Results of this preliminary study will be used to structure a larger-scale comparison of the NFP and electrolyte methods to be conducted in cooperation with established NFP teaching centers.

Introduction

Measurements of salivary and vaginal electrochemical characteristics taken with the Cue® Ovulation Predictor have been shown to be useful for prediction and confirmation of ovulation in spontaneously ovulating women (Albrecht 1987, Fernando 1985, 1988). This apparatus has been approved by the FDA and used by couples seeking to conceive since 1985. Measurements are taken using two transducers—one for daily oral readings and another for vaginal readings to be taken during the period from the Cue Peak™ until confirmation of ovulation. These electrolyte readings previously have been charted manually and interpreted by identifying three keypoints in the charts: the Cue Peak, the nadir of the vaginal readings (VR Low) and the rise from that nadir (VR Rise). The reproductive cycle keypoints are identified in the chart below:

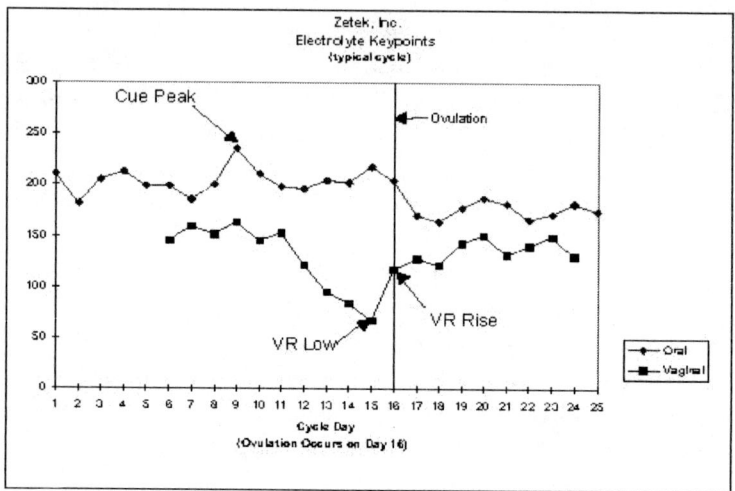

The U.S. FDA mandates that the labels for the Cue and OvaCue include the phrase "Not for Contraception." The Company and physicians recommending the instrument to infertility patients have interpreted this labeling requirement as a restriction of the Cue's use for timing of abstinence by couples seeking to avoid conception during any given cycle. However, the practice of Natural Family Planning (NFP) is in no sense limited to contraception or "avoidance" of conception. NFP principles more broadly involve control of the timing of conception and include planning to achieve conception. It is in the context of that principle that the study of the effectiveness of the Cue method for NFP use is appropriate.

The OvaCue® Fertility Monitor, a new embodiment of the Electrolyte Method™, eliminates the need for manual charting. The monitor records up to four months of oral and vaginal readings and will interpret those readings automatically. The OvaCue will reply to the inquiry "Calculate Fertility" with a fertility status indicator for that cycle day (progress bar from 1 to 7) and indicate the expected maximum fertility days for the cycle, assuming readings have been taken and the Cue Peak was found. Once the VR Low is identified, the OvaCue will also confirm that ovulation has occurred and post-ovulatory infertility has begun for the duration of that cycle. The instrument will also allow those readings to be downloaded to a computer for permanent storage and use with the OvaGraph™ software.

Four studies have been carried out in which NFP signs were compared to the manually charted Cue readings (Barrett 1985: Fazleabas 1990: Fehring 1994: Moreno, Khan-Daewood, and Goldzieher 1997). Similarly, the current study was undertaken to compare the algorithm-interpreted readings (OvaCue/OvaGraph) to several established methods of NFP. A secondary aim of the study was to develop a clearly defined protocol for use of the OvaCue system by couples wishing to avoid or postpone conception.

Materials and Methods
Subjects

Data were obtained in 24 cycles from 11 women. Subjects were recruited through referral by recognized instructors of several NFP methods and through a special NFP interest user list on the Internet. All subjects were spontaneously ovulatory and had menstrual cycles ranging in length from 24 to 36 days. After reviewing a detailed outline of the study and receiving answers to any questions, each woman submitted a signed letter of informed consent.

In order to augment testing of the automated algorithm, 29 cycles of data from an earlier study were included in this study and processed by the OvaGraph fertility software (Barrett 1985). The OvaGraph computer program contains the same data-interpretation algorithm incorporated into the OvaCue monitor. Subjects in this group had also received full information and given their informed consent.

Experimental Measurements

Subjects used the OvaCue instrument according to standard instructions, taking oral readings daily and vaginal readings on days when prompted by the device or when the algorithm indicated any level of fertility. Observations of fertility signs were recorded according to each subject's present standard NFP practice. Cervical mucus quality and quantity ("mucus"), cervical position and openness ("cervix"), and basal body temperature (BBT), when part of the subject's standard method, were recorded. The designation "sympto-thermal" was applied to those cycles in which a combination of mucus and/or cervical evaluation with use of the BBT post-ovulatory shift was used. A broad range of NFP methods was represented, with variations among centers as well as among users in format and nomenclature. However, insufficient numbers of subjects using any single method prevented inter-method comparisons.

Urine luteinizing hormone (uLH) was measured using the Lady Ovulation Tester on days identified by the OvaCue algorithm as days of maximum fertility. In the cycles from the previous study, daily 24-hour urine was collected on expected days of maximum fertility as determined by the researchers (Barrett 1985) based on the peak in Cue oral readings. These samples were analyzed for LH using standard laboratory methods. The day of peak concentration of urinary LH was taken as the day of ovulation (Wilcox et al. 1995).

Data Analysis

In conformity with previously reported procedures (Albrecht 1985), oral readings were standardized relative to the preovulatory peak in the oral readings (Cue Peak) as identified by the algorithm as a high value followed by two or more markedly lower readings. Data from the vaginal readings (VR) were standardized relative to the day of the VR Low.

The effectiveness of each approach (NFP evaluations and the OvaCue algorithm) in determining the fertility of each cycle was evaluated by comparing its identification of fertile days to the "fertile window" as defined by research performed at the National Institute of Environmental Health Sciences (Wilcox et al. 1995). Wilcox and his colleagues studied 708 cycles contributed by 221 women, and concluded that, based on the day of ovulation defined by daily uLH assays, "all conceptions resulted from intercourse that occurred during a six-day interval ending on the day of ovulation." The fertile window defined by the algorithm was taken to begin on the first day the OvaCue fertility status was >=3 bars and to end on the day the status returned to 3 bars, after days indicated maximum fertility had occurred.

An effort to impose consistency among the differing NFP reports was made by coding the descriptors. A numerical code was applied to descriptions of mucus sensation (0-3) stretchiness (0-3) type (0-2) color (0-4) and texture (0-4) and to cervix texture (0-3) os character (0-3) and position (0-3). The code zero was applied to the "least fertile" descriptor in each category, e.g., stretch code 3 indicated a spinn-barkheit of 1 inch or more, while code 1 indicated ¼ to ½ inch A code score of more than 2 in any mucus category was taken as an indicator of fertility. The BBT shift was identified retrospectively as the first day of a sustained upward shift in BBT.

Results were evaluated against the following criteria (1) days within the "fertile window" identified as infertile by the method and (2) days outside the "fertile window" identified as fertile by the method.

Results

Data were collected from 53 cycles, of which 48 were usable. Four cycles were not included in the calculations because of incomplete data, and one cycle was not used because the cycle length was beyond the definitions of the study. The LH surge was determined in 33 of the 48 useable cycles.

Results of OvaCue algorithm-interpreted data were compared to conclusions made by each of the NFP methods. For determining the end of the fertile window, the OvaCue method correlated most highly with the sympto-thermal method ($r = 0.79$), and monitoring mucus symptoms ($r = 0.74$). In all cases the OvaCue method correlated higher in determining the end of the fertile window than the beginning (Table 1).

Table 1: Correlation of OvaCue method with NFP methods

Method	Fertile Window Start	Fertile Window End
Mucus	0.58	0.74
Sympto-thermal	0.60	0.79

The methods were also compared for effectiveness in determining the beginning and end of the fertile window. The results of that comparison are shown in Table 2.

Table 2: Comparison of methods in determining the fertile window

Method	Fertile Window Start	Fertile Window End
Mucus	0.63	0.77
Sympto-Thermal	0.68	0.82
OvaCue	0.85	0.78

OvaCue and sympto-thermal data were then analyzed to determine the number of days in the fertile window that were interpreted as infertile (case 1) and the number of days outside the fertile window that were interpreted as fertile (case 2). Assuming an avoidance posture, the days in case 1 would be those that could lead to unintended pregnancy and in case 2 as those where abstinence was recommended erroneously. Percentages were calculated based on the total number of days in the fertile window (33 cycles x 6 days in fertile window = 198 fertility days). Percentages for Case 2 were not calculated as total cycle days outside the fertile window since data from all cycles was not available. Results of the analysis are in Table 3.

Table 3: Effectiveness of methods for NFP use

Method	Case 1	% Effective	Case 2
OvaCue Algorithm	2 days	98.99	92 days
Sympto-Thermal	25 days	87.38	148 days

Using an OvaCue conception avoidance protocol of the first fertility sign (bar = 3) to the last high fertility (bar = 5), 2 fertile days out of 198 were mis-identified as infertile. Using sympto-thermal methods, 25 fertile days were mis-identified as infertile. In the same cycles, unnecessary avoidance occurred on 61% more days using sympto-thermal methods than the OvaCue method (148 vs. 92).

Discussion

Participants reported that both the OvaCue and NFP methods were used without difficulty. After becoming acquainted with the basic menus and setup procedure of the OvaCue, users reported finding the OvaCue easy to use and understand. Oral readings are only required during the follicular and ovulatory phases of the cycle. Nevertheless, most subjects preferred developing the habit of taking an oral reading daily. Subjects reported that use of the vaginal sensor for a few days each cycle was not burdensome.

Self-evaluation of fertility signs using NFP methods is simple, easy-to-learn, and effective. While sufficient samples for statistical comparison between methods was not available, it was observed that many of the more experienced self-observers abstract the most relevant components from the NFP method initially learned. This was an interesting result of not specifying any particular method for use by these women. Some omitted BBT; some knew they did not need to begin observations before a certain cycle day; many did not use cervical characteristics; most discontinued observations once the fertile window had been recognized.

Although NFP methods have long been known to be effective, there are circumstances when a more objective means of evaluation is desirable. These would include women with irregular cycle lengths and those who incur fertility signs that are not readily apparent. Objective evaluation would be beneficial to those beginning NFP practice, and those desiring additional confidence in using NFP methods. Additionally, certain couples may find the use of an automated fertility-monitoring device attractive. It was determined that because the methods do not conflict from a procedural standpoint, the OvaCue could be used in conjunction with NFP methods without interference.

A benefit of this study has been to define more closely the protocol for any further investigations of the OvaCue/OvaGraph. In the future, a series of studies of which each cohort uses the same NFP method of self-observation would allow examination of the NFP method in relation to the Zetek electrolyte method.

Conclusions

Correlation among the OvaCue method and various NFP methods were varied. The closest relation exists between the Sympto-thermal method and the OvaCue method, with the methods being closer in determining the end of the fertile period and differing more in defining its beginning. Correlations of each method with the fertile window as defined by the LH surge led to the conclusion that the methods were similarly effective at determining the end of the fertile window, but the OvaCue was more effective for determining the beginning of the fertile window.

Based on the criteria of having no fertile days identified as infertile, the OvaCue algorithm correctly processed 46 of 48 cycles (96%). This result corresponds to conclusions made in earlier studies (Fernando 1988).

In this study, the OvaCue/OvaGraph algorithm was effective at identifying the fertile window and has potential to be used as an adjunctive device in the learning and use of NFP methods. Although a limited number of cycles were evaluated in this study, the initially positive results warrant a larger study. Goals for a future study would include further definition of the protocol for achieving or avoiding conception as well as to evaluate the efficacy of the automated method.

Improved data quality can be expected from coordinating the study participants through a centralized location. A requirement that participants use the same NFP method and be consistent and diligent in charting techniques and data reporting could also provide methodology improvements. In the future, Zetek intends to complete a large-scale study in cooperation with one or more established NFP teaching centers in order to define more fully the efficacy and applications of the Electrolyte Method.

Bibliography

Albrecht, B.H., Fernando, R.S., Regas, J., and Betz, G. 1985. "A new method for predicting and confirming ovulation." *Fertility and Sterility* 44:200.

Barrett, K. 1985. *An Interim report on the Cue® ovulation predictor, a natural family planning perspective.* Fourth National and International Symposium on Natural Family Planning, Washington D.C., November 3-6, 1985.

Fazleabas, A.T., Segraves, M.M., and Khan-Dawood, F.S. 1990. "Evaluation of salivary and vaginal electrical measurements for determination of the time of ovulation." *International Journal of Fertility* 35(2):106.

Fehring, R.J. 1996. "A Comparison of the ovulation method with the CUE ovulation predictor in determining the fertile period." *Journal of the American Academy of Nurse Practitioners*, 8(10):461-466.

Fernando, R.S. 1988. Saliva and cervical mucus monitor to define ovulation, SBIR Phase II Report to the National Institutes of Health (Grant Number: 2 R44 HD20222-02)

Fernando, R.S., Regas, J., and Betz, G. 1988. "Ovulation prediction and detection with the CUE® ovulation predictor." *Human Reproduction 3:*419.

Fernando, R.S., Regas, J., and Betz, G. 1987. "Prediction of ovulation with the use of oral and vaginal electrical measurements during treatment with clomiphene citrate." *Fertility and Sterility* 47:409.

Moreno, J., Khan-Daewood, F.S., and Goldzieher, J.W. 1997. "Natural Family Planning: Suitability of the Cue method for defining the time of Ovulation." *Contraception* 55:233-237.

Wilcox, A.J., Weinberg, C.R., and Baird, D.D. 1995. "Timing of sexual intercourse in relation to ovulation: effects on the probability of conception, survival of the pregnancy, and sex of the baby." *New England Journal of Medicine* 333 (23) 1517.

Response to "Preliminary Comparison of Algorithm—Interpreted Fertility Moniter Readings with Established NFP methods"

Barbara Savinetti–Rose, R.N., M.S.N.
Philadelphia NFP Network

Changes in the electrolytes of salivary and vaginal fluids have been shown to signal the onset and completion of the ovulatory process. Previous studies of the electrolyte method and its associated use of technology (here the OvaCue Fertility Monitor) have the approval of the FDA to assist couples in achieving pregnancy.

The authors' intent in this study was to see how information from the OvaCue Fertility Monitor (OvaCue) could be compared to the physiological signs of standard NFP methods in assisting couples planning to postpone or avoid pregnancy. While there are some significant flaws in this study's design, the researchers are to be commended for attempting to demonstrate the OvaCue's accuracy in concert with established methods of NFP. This is aptly called a *preliminary* study of how the OvaCue and NFP methods rated in identifying the fertile phase of a woman's cycle when compared to the urinary luitenizing hormone (LH) surge, the standard in identifying ovulation established by Wilcox et al. in 1995.

Small sample size

It is unfortunate that the authors did not recruit more subjects for this study. While they admitted they did not have enough data and actually supplemented with 29 cycles from an earlier study, the number of menstrual cycles evaluated was an extremely minimal total of 48. This small sample size makes it difficult to draw any conclusions. Most other comparison studies in NFP evaluate hundreds and thousands of women's cycles.

Confusion of NFP methodology

The authors have stated that they wished to compare the OvaCue with three established methods of NFP, namely "mucus, cervix, and STM." In utilizing the term "mucus method" it is assumed that the women were practicing some form of the ovulation method. In describing a sympto-thermal method (STM), the biological markers are primarily mucus and temperature. It is not correct to state that there is an established NFP method called the "cervix method."

There is no formal rule using the cervix alone as a biological marker for fertility. There are only anecdotal reports by some women, particularly those in pre-menopause, that the cervix position change is a reliable sign for the end of the fertile phase. For these women, the fourth day of a closing cervix, cross-checked by the elevated temperature rise, indicates the end of their fertile phase. To date, there have been no studies conducted on a cervix-only rule and therefore it is incorrect to define it as an "established method" of NFP (Parenteau-Carreau and Infante-Rivard, 1988). Perhaps the researchers here are confusing NFP methods with biological markers of fertility. This may be the reason that the data in the tables identified as cervix method do not correlate very well.

Identifying the beginning and end of the fertile phase

By declaring the day of the urinary LH surge as day of ovulation and identifying the prior five days as fertile, the authors compared the OvaCue's start of the fertile period with that of the NFP methods. The question first arises, at what point did the subjects begin testing their urine for LH? Through personal communication with the researchers, it was clarified that the days of maximum fertility as indicated by the OvaCue were days that the subjects commenced their urinary testing. However "in cycles where the oral readings were in the high range, referred to in the study, subjects were to institute LH testing when fertility was indicated by either the OvaCue or their NFP observations. In the supplementary cycles, LH testing was scheduled by the investigator based on the Cue Peak." (P. Regas, personal communication, April 16, 2002)

The authors of this study concluded that the OvaCue was more accurate in determining the start of fertile phase than all three NFP methods. What we do not know however, is what specific rules the subjects were following in identifying the start of their fertile phase by their NFP method. While there is consensus among ovulation method users that the first day of mucus detection is the beginning of the fertile phase, there isn't any specific consensus among STM users regarding the start of the fertile phase. In the STM as taught by Couple to Couple League, the beginning of the fertile phase can be the first day of mucus detection, otherwise known as the "last dry day rule," provided there is a minimum five day mucus patch. Other rules are, "clinical experience," "Doering," and the "21/20 day rule" (Kippley, 1997, p. 182). The start of the fertile window in the cervix method does not exist as the cervix is only used as a biological marker to determine the end of the fertile phase by the rules established in the anecdotal reports.

The authors described how the OvaCue and the STM method were closer in determining the end of the fertile phase than the other NFP methods. Here again, there is no evidence that the participants were following the same rules. For example, the end of the fertile period for subjects following ovulation methods could be defined as either the morning of the fourth day past the peak mucus symptom or the evening of the fourth day past the peak mucus symptom. Identifying the end of the fertile phase in STM can also be variable because it will depend on the strength of the thermal shift. In the CCL definitions, the strengths of the shifts are classified as overall, strong or full. Study participants who are identifying the end of their fertile phase using a strong thermal shift will quite possibly resume sexual activity later than those who identify the end of their fertile phase utilizing an overall thermal shift. The end of the fertile phase by the cervix method is suspect, as we do not know if the subjects are cross-checking with temperature and there is no information as to the strength of that thermal shift before they declare themselves infertile. Obviously, the authors must have realized this error when they collected the data as they have admitted that in future studies "methodology improvements could also be made by requiring that participants use the same NFP method and be consistent and diligent in charting techniques and data reporting"

Determining the accuracy of the fertile window to postpone pregnancy

A concern when postponing or avoiding pregnancy for couples practicing NFP is that they may mistakenly consider a day in the fertile window to be an infertile day, thereby engaging in sexual activity that would lead to a pregnancy. In this regard, the authors report the OvaCue was far more reliable than the STM. The device had reported only 2 out of 193 days of mistaken infertility as compared to 25 days out of 193 days of mistaken infertility using the STM. Here again it is not known which rules the participants were following when they declared that they were practicing a STM. The finding of the OvaCue's accuracy in identifying the fertile window is not too surprising, given the fact that the device has been shown in previous studies to be close enough to ovulation to be used for scheduling inseminations and other procedures.

The search for an objective measure of fertility for special circumstances

While the authors declared that a more obective measure of fertility might be helpful when there are ovulatory disorders, irregular cycle lengths, or vague fertility signs, they did not set out to prove the device's effectiveness in this area. All of the subjects in this study were described as normal and healthy with cycle lengths of 24 to 36 days. What we don't have is any information as to the motivation of these couples. Did they volunteer for this study in the hope that they would obtain a more objective measure of their own fertility? Were they experiencing vague or confusing fertility signs? Were they looking for a gadget that could help them more accurately determine their fertile phase and thereby reduce their anxiety? If they were experiencing confusion it might explain some of the data in the last table that reports there being unnecessary avoidance occurring more often in practicing a STM compared to that of the OvaCue (148 vs. 92).

Conclusion

As the authors suggest, a device with a proven record of reliability with regard to the identification of the fertile phase may have a future as an "adjunctive device in the learning and use of NFP methods." To that end, this author agrees. It is however, premature to suggest that it could be used alone as a method of family planning or that it is somehow superior to the current established NFP methods that rely on the identification and interpretation of a woman's physiological signs.

It is hoped that the OvaCue's growing market will affect the public's perception of NFP as a reliable method of birth regulation. Those who are unconvinced that the natural methods are effective may reconsider when they see how this latest device provides additional data to determine a woman's fertile phase. Couples in Western nations may not mind the added expense of the OvaCue and may come to trust its accuracy in identifying the fertile phase when planning periods of abstinence.

Bibliography

Kippley, John F. and Kippley, Sheila K. 1997. *The Art of Natural Family Planning*, 4 th edition. Cincinnati: The Couple to Couple League.

Parenteau-Carreau, S. and Infante-Rivard, C. 1988. "Self-palpation to assess cervical changes in relation to mucus and temperature." *International Journal of Fertility*. Supplement:10-16.

Wilcox, A.J., Weinberg, C.R., and Baird, D.D. 1995. "Timing of sexual intercourse in relation to ovulation. Effects on the probability of conception, survival of the pregnancy, and the sex of the baby." *New England Journal of Medicine* 333 (23):1517-1521.

Undergirding Abstinence within a Sexuality Education Program
An Analysis of Outcome Data of the 1999-2001 Teen Star Program

Hanna Klaus, M.D.
Mary Nora Dennehy
Jean Turnbull

Summary

The efficacy of the Teen STAR Program, a proactive educational program in human sexuality to undergird virginity and/or facilitate a return to chastity has been reported previously. The 1999-2001 cohorts are similar to the previously reported cohorts. The 8-month program joins experiential learning of fertility signs to a developmental didactic curriculum plus regular teacher student interaction. Our U.S. study population from 5 sites consisted of 822 males aged 12-17 years; 71 were sexually active, 42 virgins (5.5%) transitioned to sexual activity, while 55 (49%) discontinued activity. Of 496 females aged 12-16 years 16 (3.2%) were sexually active, before the program, 14 (2.9%) transitioned while 16 (53%) discontinued activity. The rate of discontinuation was approximately double of that among the general population: 53 vs. 26 % for females, 49 vs. 27% for males.

Responses were stratified by early, middle and late adolescence and tabulated by virgin/non-virgin status. Both virgins and non-virgins identified chastity, the consequences of sex: unwanted pregnancy and STDs, and self-knowledge as the most important thing(s) they learned and remembered about the program. The previously validated Likert scale measured behavioral parameters: speaking about the program with parents, with friends, greater control of emotions, greater empathy with others, overall helpfulness of the program and reasons for maintaining or returning to chastity. In middle and late adolescence non-virgins generally presented at the lower end of the scale in all parameters, lending support to Erikson's theory of identity foreclosure or at least delay as a result of participation in adult tasks before emotional maturity has been reached, while early adolescents were equally enthusiastic, and predominantly returned to chastity. The fact that at least half of locus of control responses indicated an internal locus may indicate progress toward growing up. Failure to discontinue intercourse was associated with contraceptive use by 72% of the males and 43% of the females.

Conclusion

Tracking of fertility patterns joined to discussion of their meaning correlates positively with maintaining virginity as well as a return to chastity. The overall 50% discontinuation rate exceeds that of the general population and can be an important tool for prevention of STD and premarital pregnancy.

Introduction

Despite recent declining rates in adolescent pregnancy in this country, more than four in ten teenage girls still get pregnant at least once before age 20. About two-thirds of all students have sex before graduating from high school, potentially exposing themselves to STDs. And one in four sexually experienced teens do contract an STD each year, some of which are incurable, including HIV, which is terminal or at least life-threatening (Kirby 2001).

Yet the percentage of adolescents primarily or secondarily abstinent may be increased at least in the short term by well-designed programs adeptly implemented in a community of receptive teens. Parental involvement, solid theoretical grounding, reinforcement of appropriate social norms, as well as teaching the interpersonal skills necessary to remain abstinent appear promising for program success (Thomas 2000).

The concept of abstinence embraces both primary abstinence; that is, refraining from sexual intercourse by an individual who has never experienced it, and secondary abstinence, the discontinuation of sexual intercourse by those already experienced (Thomas 2000). It is believed that abstinence provides buffering from the psychosocial and emotional harm that result from premature sexual relationships (Orr et al. 1991; Billy et al. 1988).

A University of Minnesota statewide survey of adolescent health that included 26,023 students in Grades 7 through 12 in 1988 found some interesting emotional correlates to delayed sexual intercourse. Among adolescent females aged 13-14 years, those with lower symptoms of depression were less likely to have initiated intercourse. Male youth who were concerned about issues within their communities (alcohol, drugs, violence, and hunger) were less likely than peers to initiate early sexual intercourse. Females who likewise expressed social concerns were also less likely to have early intercourse than peers. The same was true, but less strong, for those who reported themselves as more religious. The likelihood that females or males with higher school performance would have initiated sexual intercourse was more than half that of peers with lower school performance (Lammers et al. 2000).

Several abstinence-based programs, as well as my own experience, suggest that adolescents are neither able to understand fully the implications of their sexual experimentation, nor to deal with the consequences of such activity. According to the work of Marion Howard at Grady Memorial Hospital in Atlanta, Georgia, the needs that teenagers seek to meet through sexual intercourse could best be met in other ways. Moreover, teens are often pressured into sexual behaviors in which they do not want to engage. They require preparatory awareness of sexual pressures and the skills needed to resist them (Howard and McCabe 1990).

In one poll, 12 to 17 year olds identified the pressure to have sex as the number one threat to their well being (Worldwide 1994). A poll of 1,000 adolescent girls in an adolescent clinic in Atlanta found the topic most desired to have discussed, 84% of those polled, was how to say no to a boyfriend's request to have sex without losing the boyfriend or hurting his feelings (Howard and McCabe 1990).

Implications can also be found in a number of studies for consideration in developing prevention of high-risk behaviors among adolescents. For example, if peers are a significant influence, efforts to reduce adolescent pregnancy, AIDS, and other STDs should account for peers in prevention strategies. Providing adolescents with roles in prevention efforts may increase the likelihood that peer reinforcement will work in prosocial ways (DiBlasio and Benda 1990).

Increasing education, awareness, and involvement of parents in sexual issues of their children may be effective, as adolescents considered positive and negative consequences of their actions in the light of parental reactions. For example, high school students in the DiBlasio and Benda study (1990) reported that greater supervision and discipline by parents would reduce their sexual frequency. Additionally, creation of a normative climate by youths and adults that makes it popular to postpone sexual intercourse until adulthood may influence adolescents in the direction of attitudes and beliefs against early sexual involvement.

Reduction or prevention of teenage pregnancies is a high priority due to the high risk of physical, emotional, and social problems for mother and child. The more prevalent approach is the provision of contraception. The continuing high rates of both teen pregnancy and abortion, however, testify to the less than universal efficacy of the contraceptive approach. The effectiveness of an oral contraceptive is high, but it appears that in spite of powerful public information campaigns, teenagers do not accept them, or fail to use them consistently (Klaus et al. 1987).

My seven year experience of teaching prenatal and parenting education to a group of pregnant and/or parenting teens at an alternate school for low income high school dropouts or truants gave me personal experience of this (MND). Most of the young women in these classes had experienced physical and/or emotional side effects or failure from various contraceptives, with little understanding or patience from the medical community or their partners.

Neither the provision of contraception nor the exhortation to preserve chastity serves adolescents' need to integrate their now-present biological capacity to procreate into their operational self-concepts. The Teen STAR program utilizing experiential learning about fertility to facilitate the integration of biologic maturity with adolescent emotions, cognition, capacity, life goals and behavior was developed to address this need (Klaus et al.1988).

Contraception dichotomizes sex and procreation, thus facilitating fragmented, often solely or largely genital, relationships, which do not lead to growth. While teens are often exposed to exhortation to moral (chaste) behavior, many have not yet reached the level of personal integration to accept this teaching, even when disposed to do so, because they are immersed in the adolescent personality task of establishing their ego identity. This requires at least a theoretical distancing from the "parental ego" in order to discover which values are their own, and which are passively incorporated from their parent(s). These adolescents cannot "hear" adults when they say that genital union can only have its full meaning within marriage, because they still need to master the preliminary adolescent personality tasks. A high priority for teens is to understand their sexuality as well as their procreative capacity. It seems that until youth can "own" their fertility more than just intellectually they cannot integrate their sexuality and become more mature. Only after coming to terms with the fact that one is now biologically capable of becoming a mother or a father, can awareness of this capacity be integrated into choices about present behaviors that are consistent with future life goals (Klaus 1988).

The original Teen STAR pilot program was designed to discover whether young women could be taught to recognize their fertility patterns by mucus self-detection, to monitor the effect of understanding their fertility on their sexual behavior in the context of gender-specific value-oriented curricula, and to monitor the effect of parental involvement on client continuation and behavior (Klaus 1988).

It has been my experience in working with adolescent girls most of my professional life that even those who intellectually accept sexual abstinence as a value, without further instruction, they are less likely to maintain this stance under pressure. A knowledge and experience of charting their own fertility patterns, the cyclic rise and fall of hormones with their effect on one's moods, plus concrete ways of responding to these emotional changes and pressures is empowering to the adolescent girl and reinforcing of abstinence outside of a totally committed relationship. I have also learned that instruction in fertility awareness enables the adolescent to come to a new and deeper understanding of what it means to be a woman. Developing a healthy feminine identity and full acceptance of ones' sexuality is part of adolescent development.

Estrogens release endorphins, making us feel good, even-tempered and outgoing. After ovulation, the metabolite of progesterone, (allopregnanolone) is anxiolytic, that is, it releases anxiety (Rapkin et al.

1997). Women become more inward looking and introspective, arty. (We often hear from parents of adolescent girls complain about how much time their daughters spend in their rooms, more than likely during the progesterone phase of their cycle.)

When both estrogen and progesterone drop, the low level of androgen in women can become dominant. Ordinarily, the female level of testosterone is one-tenth of what it is in the male. Testosterone, generally associated with energy and aggression in the male, becomes apparent three or four days before the menstrual period in women. At this time she is more apt to become impatient or have a short fuse, as teens are likely to report. For example, the behavior of a younger sibling well tolerated during most of the cycle can become an irritant at this time. This phase can be expressed inwardly as depression or outwardly as aggression.

Does this mean that the adolescent girl or woman is a victim of her hormones? Not if she is aware of her cycling hormones and their influence on her moods. She can be challenged to decide how they will affect her behavior, putting her in charge. Likewise, many adolescent girls can feel a lack of control about menstruation and its timing. With an appreciation of fertility awareness, she can learn when to predict it, giving her a feeling of being more in control.

Teens also learn the effect of hormones as well as other factors on their sexual desire. As one girl explained to me, "I almost went all the way but stopped as I remembered what you said, 'It's not true love; it's the hormones.'" I don't recall using those exact words, but the young woman got the message correctly.

Being as self invested as teens are, this knowledge of factors involved in their emotional state proves of great interest to adolescent girls, and boys I might add. Some girls may even be attracted to Teen STAR because of the psychological self-knowledge involved. Once into the program, however, they appreciate this information but experience and learn so much more in the process.

Other areas covered in the Teen Star curriculum include:
1) Psychosexual differences between men and women
2) Dating – boy/girl relationships – the purpose of dating, appropriate dating behavior, including assertive refusal techniques
3) Evaluating sexual attitudes presented on TV & other media

4) STDs
5) Consequences of premarital sex
6) The meaning of a totally committed relationship.

Methodology

In an effort to determine the effect of premature intercourse on the psychological maturation of adolescents, outcome data from anonymous exit questionnaires from the 1998-2001 Teen STAR programs in the U.S. were analyzed. Responses of 496 female and 822 male subjects were grouped by gender, virgin/non-virgin status, and level of psychosexual development; i.e., early adolescence – 11 to 13 years of age, middle adolescence – 14 to 15 years of age, and late adolescence – 16 to 17 years of age. Non-virgins represented only 10–13 % of the study groups. (Tables 1A and 1B)

Results

There were considerable differences in the responses of virgins and non-virgins across all three groups:

1) Female and male virgins in middle adolescence anticipated future abstinence more frequently than non-virgins. In late adolescence, males had no expectations, while 2/3 of females were hopeful. (Tables 2A and 2B).

2) All early adolescents gained on the question of greater control of emotions, while the gain was higher among virgins than non-virgins. (Tables 3A and 3B)

3) Early adolescent non-virgin females and middle adolescent non-virgin males lagged behind other groups on empathy with others. (Tables 4A and 4B)

4) Early and middle virgin females rated the program higher for over-all helpfulness. (Tables 5A and 5B)

5) About half of early and mid-adolescent males, whether virgin or not, spoke with their parents about the program, other than to request permission to participate, while about one third of other male groups did so. More early and late adolescent female virgins talked with their parents about the program than did female non-virgins. A higher percentage of middle adolescent female non-virgins, although small in actual number, spoke with their parents about the program

than did the percentage of middle adolescent female virgins. (Tables 6A and 6B)

6) A greater percentage of middle and late adolescent virgin males spoke with their friends about the program while a greater percentage of early adolescent male non-virgins spoke with their friends about the program than did early adolescent male virgins. The opposite was true for females, with more early adolescent virgins and a greater percentage, though small in actual number, middle and late female non-virgins talked to their friends about the program. (Tables 7A and 7B)

7) Virgins of course had higher response rates for reasons for remaining (or returning to) abstinence than non-virgins; they also had a much higher rate of responses which reflected an internal locus of control, indicating movement toward maturity. (Tables 8A&B) Table 9 identifies the questions and their loci. There was little difference between what students remembered most from the course (Tables 10 A and 10B) and what they considered most important. (Tables 11A and 11B) All listed chastity, consequences of sex and self-knowledge. Girls added knowledge of their fertility cycle.

Non-virgins presented at the lower end of the scale in all parameters, lending support to Erikson's theory of identity foreclosure or at least delay, as a result of participation in adult tasks before emotional maturity has been reached. Failure to discontinue intercourse was linked to contraceptive use in all three age groups. This was more pronounced among males (72%) than females (43%). (Table 12)

Conclusion

Tracking of fertility patterns joined to discussion of their meaning correlates positively with maintaining virginity as well as a return to chastity. The high level of continuing virginity, as well as the overall 50% discontinuation of sexual activity exceeds that of the general population and can be an important tool for prevention of STDs and premarital pregnancy (Klaus 2001).

Tables

Table 1: Sexual Activity and Contraceptive Use, TEEN STAR 1999-2001, USA / Youth Risk Behavior Survey - 1999

Table 1A: Males

Age	Total N	Active Prior N(%)	Began during N(%)	Contrac. "Nearly always" N(%)	Discontinued interc. N(%)	Active prior %	Curr. Active %	Curr.* Abstin't %
11	8	2(25)	1(15)	-	2(66)	age<13		
12	33	1(3)	1(3.1)	-	2(100)	[14.2]		
13	48	4(8.3)	5(11.3)	-	4(44)	-		
14	306	29(9.4)	16(5.7)	39(72)	27(49)	44.5	29.1	31.3
15	392	32(8.8)	16(4.4)	39(50)	18(38)	51.1	33.9	29.2
16	34	3(8.8)	2(64)	-	1(20)	51.4	35.4	28.6
17	1	0	1(100)	-	1(100)	63.9	48.1	22.0
Total	822	71(9.40)	41(5.4)	78(70)	39(35)			

Table 1B: Females

Age	Total N	Active Prior N(%)	Began during N(%)	Contrac. "Nearly always" N(%)	Discontinued interc. N(%)	Active prior %	Curr. Active %	Curr. Abstin't %
11	5	0	0					
12	36	1(2.7)	2(5.7)	1(33)	1(33)	age<13		
13	68	3(4.4)	2(3.0)	0	2(40)	[4.4]		
14	189	4(2.1)	3(1.6)	1(16)	5(71)	32.5	24.0	26.7
15	187	7(3.7)	5(2.7)	9(60)	6(50)	42.6	32.0	24.8
16	11	1(9)	2(20)	2(33)	2(33)	53.8	39.5	26.5
Total	496	16(3.2)	14(2.9)	13(43)	19(63)			

Table 2: Positive influence of fertility awareness perceived on sexual behavior—determined, or less likely to have sex before marriage.

Table 2A: Males

Age	Virgin		Non-Virgin	
	Number	Percent	Number	Percent
11-13 years	75	65%	14	50%
14-15 years	594	75%	103	50%
16 years	29	86%	6	50%

Table 2B: Females

Age	Virgin		Non-Virgin	
	Number	Percent	Number	Percent
11-13 years	101	72%	8	50%
14-15 years	354	84%	22	64%
16 years	8	37%	3	66%

Table 3: Greater Control of Emotions Perceived by (%).

Table 3A: Males

Age	Virgin		Non-Virgin	
	Number	Percent	Number	Percent
11-13 years	75	71%	14	71%
14-15 years	594	68%	103	60%
16 years	29	72%	6	83%

Table 3B: Females

Age	Virgin		Non-Virgin	
	Number	Percent	Number	Percent
11-13 years	101	82%	8	62%
14-15 years	354	71%	22	68%
16 years	8	50%	3	66%

Table 4: Greater Empathy with Others Perceived by (%).

Table 4A: Males

Age	Virgin		Non-Virgin	
	Number	Percent	Number	Percent
11-13 years	75	67%	14	50%
14-15 years	594	77%	103	75%
16 years	29	79%	6	33%

Table 4B: Females

Age	Virgin		Non-Virgin	
	Number	Percent	Number	Percent
11-13 years	101	83%	8	75%
14-15 years	354	79%	22	77%
16 years	8	62%	3	100%

Table 5: Overall Helpfulness of Program.

Table 5A: Males

Age	Virgin		Non-Virgin	
	Number	Percent	Number	Percent
11-13 years	75	81%	14	93%
14-15 years	594	86%	103	74%
16 years	29	83%	6	50%

Table 5B: Females

Age	Virgin		Non-Virgin	
	Number	Percent	Number	Percent
11-13 years	101	90%	8	77%
14-15 years	354	88%	22	77%
16 years	8	77%	3	100%

Table 6: Talked with Parents about Program.

Table 6A: Males

Age	Virgin		Non-Virgin	
	Number	Percent	Number	Percent
11-13 years	75	55%	14	36%
14-15 years	594	49%	103	29%
16 years	29	31%	6	33%

Table 6B: Females

Age	Virgin		Non-Virgin	
	Number	Percent	Number	Percent
11-13 years	101	70%	8	50%
14-15 years	354	50%	22	64%
16 years	8	55%	3	33%

Table 7: Talked with Friends about Program.

Table 7A: Males

Age	Virgin		Non-Virgin	
	Number	Percent	Number	Percent
11-13 years	75	58%	14	64%
14-15 years	594	68%	103	63%
16 years	29	86%	6	66%

Table 7B: Females

Age	Virgin		Non-Virgin	
	Number	Percent	Number	Percent
11-13 years	101	82%	8	75%
14-15 years	354	85%	22	86%
16 years	8	55%	3	66%

Table 8: Reasons for Remaining Chaste (Virgin) or Returning to Chastity (Non-Virgin)*
by External and Internal Locus of control: N = %.

Table 8A: Males*				
Age	Virgin		Non-Virgin	
	External	Internal	External	Internal
11-13 years	45 = 60%	33 = 44%	4 = 29%	1 = 7%
14-15 years	475 = 80%	407 = 69%	25 = 24%	9 = 9%
16 years	26 = 90%	14 = 48%	2 = 33%	-

Table 8B: Females*				
Age	Virgin		Non-Virgin	
	Number	Percent	Number	Percent
11-13 years	70 = 69%	67 = 66%	1 = 12%	1 = 12%
14-15 years	304 = 86%	299 = 84%	6 = 27%	5 = 22%
16 years	7 = 87%	3 = 33%	1 = 33%	1 = 33%

* Many responses were incomplete mostly at the student's choice, but also because of incomplete copying of tests by one large co-ed school.

Table 9: Reasons for not having sex identified by locus of control (I = internal locus, E = external locus)

"If you haven't had sex, or if you are abstaining from any further sexual contact, which of the following reasons for NOT having sex are important to you? (Check all that apply.) "

01. It is against my religious beliefs. — E
02. It just doesn't seem like a very smart thing to do. — I
03. I don't want to face the problems of an unwanted pregnancy. — E
04. I don't want to get AIDS or some other sexually transmitted disease. — E
05. I haven't found the right person. — I
06. I haven't had an opportunity. — I
07. I wouldn't feel comfortable doing it. — I
08. I feel it's morally wrong. — E
09. I don't feel I'm ready. — I
10. I don't want to disappoint my parents. — E
11. I don't want to be used or taken advantage of. — I
12. Other:

Table 10: Most frequently remembered topics

	Table 10A: Males	
Age	Virgin	Non-Virgin
11-13 years	"Other." Chastity. Unwanted pregnancy as consequence of sex. Contraception. Self-knowledge. Videos. N = 75	"Other." Self-knowledge. Videos. Chastity. N = 14
14-15 years	Self-knowledge. Unwanted pregnancy as consequence of sex. STD's. Videos. N = 594	"Other." Negative comment. STD's. Unwanted pregnancy as consequence of sex. N = 103
16 years	Unwanted pregnancy as consequence of sex. The teacher. Videos. STD's. N = 29	"other" Cycle. STD's. Self-knowledge. Negative Comment. N = 6

	Table 10B: Females	
Age	Virgin	Non-Virgin
11-13 years	"Other." Self-knowledge. -the Cycle. Chastity. N = 101	Cycle. Self-knowledge. Chastity. N = 8
14-15 years	Unwanted pregnancy as consequence of sex. Speakers. STD's. Abortion. "Other." N = 354	Unwanted pregnancy as consequence of sex. "Other." STD's. Abortion. Speakers. N = 22
16 years	"Other." Videos. N = 8	STD's. Unwanted pregnancy as consequence of sex. N = 3

Table 11: Most frequently remembered topics

	Table 11A: Males	
Age	Virgin	Non-Virgin
11-13 years	"Other." Chastity. "Other." STD's. Abortion. N = 75	Chastity. Unwanted pregnancy as consequence of sex. HIV/AIDS. Self-knowledge. N = 14
14-15 years	Chastity. "Other." STD's. Self-knowledge. Unwanted pregnancy as consequence of sex. N = 594	"Other." Chastity. STD's. Self-knowledge. Negative comment. N = 103
16 years	Chastity. Unwanted pregnancy as consequence of sex. STD's. Abortion. N = 29	STD's. Self-knowledge. Chastity. Negative Comment. N = 6

	Table 11B: Females	
Age	Virgin	Non-Virgin
11-13 years	"Other." Responsibility/respect/consequences of choices. Self-knowledge. N = 101	Cycle. Self-Knowledge. STD's. Unwanted pregnancy as consequence of sex. Videos. Chastity. N = 8
14-15 years	Chastity. Unwanted pregnancy as consequence of sex. "Other." STD's. N = 354	"Other." Unwanted pregnancy as consequence of sex. STD's. N = 22
16 years	"Other." Abortion. STD's. HIV/AIDS. Contraception. N = 8	Chastity. Unwanted pregnancy as consequence of sex. N = 3

Table 12: Continued Sex Activity vs. Use of Contraception

Table 12A: Males		
Male 11-13 6 continued	Total 14 2 used always or most of the time	= 33%
Male 14-15 57 continued	Total 103 43 used always or most of the time 1 didn't answer	= 75%
Male 16-17 5 continued	Total 6 4 used always or most of the time	= 80%

Of the 68 males who continued sexual activity 49 (72%) also continued to use contraception

Table 12B: Females		
Female 11-13 5 continued	Total 8 2 used always or most of the time	= 40%
Female 14-15 10 continued	Total 22 4 used always or most of the time 1 didn't answer	= 40%
Female 1 1 continued	Total 3 1 used always or most of the time	= 100%

Of the 17 females who continued sexual activity 7 (43%) also continued to use contraception

Bibliography

Billy, J., Landale, N., Grady, W., and Zimmerle, D. 1988. "Effects of sexual activity on adolescent social and psychological development." *Soc Psychology Quarterly* 51:190-212.

DiBlasio, F.A., and Benda, B.B. 1990. "Adolescent Sexual Behavior: Multivariate Analysis of a Social Learning Model." *Journal of Adolescent Research* 5:414-429.

Howard, M., and McCabe, J.B. 1990. "Helping teenagers postpone sexual involvement." *Family Planning Perspectives* 20:21-6.

Kirby, D. May 2001. *Emerging Answers: Research Findings on Programs to Reduce Teen Pregnancy.* National Campaign to Prevent Teen Pregnancy. Washington, DC.

Klaus, H. 2001. *Teen STAR News.* Bethesda, MD.

Klaus, H., Fagan, M.U., Bryant, M.L., Dausman, S., Dennehy, N., Begley, M., Monmonier, H., & Martin, J.L. "Teen STAR: *S*exuality *T*eaching in the Context of *A*dult *R*esponsibility." Regier, G. Ed. 1988. *Values and Public Policy.* Washington, D.C.: Family Research Council.

Klaus, H., Bryan, L.M., Bryant, M.L., Fagan, M.U., Harrigan, M.B., and Kearns, F. 1987. "Fertility Awareness/Natural Family Planning for Adolescents and their Families: Report of Multi-site Pilot Project. *International Journal of Adolescent Medicine & Health* 3:2:101-119.

Lammers, C., Ireland, M., Resnick, M., & Blum, R. 2000. "Influences on Adolescents' Decision to Postpone Onset of Sexual Intercourse: A survival Analysis of Virginity among Youths Aged 13 to 18 Years." *Journal of Adolescent Health* 26:42-48.

Orr, D., Bexter, M., & Ingersoll, G. 1991. "Premature sexual activity as an indicator of psychosocial risk." *Pediatrics* 87: 41-7.

Thomas, M.H. 2000. "Abstinence-Based Programs for Prevention of Adolescent Pregnancies: A Review." *Journal of Adolescent Health* 26:5-17.

Worldwide, Roper Starch. 1994. Teens Talk About Sex: Adolescent Sexuality in the 90s. New York: Sexuality Information and Education Council of the United States.

Youth Risk Behavior Survey, United States. 1999. Centers for Disease Control, DHHS.

Acknowledgements:

Program data were contributed by: Liz Heyne and Bertha Moreno, Dallas, TX:; Mary Ann Fennell and her group from Fairfax, VA;, Jean Turnbull, Philadelphia, PA; Tom and Chiquita Seesan, Massillon OH; Lorraine Leonard, St. Andrew's, Andrews AFB, MD. Irene Arevalo performed data entry and analysis.

An earlier version of this paper was presented at the 2001 Teen Pregnancy Prevention Conference, Pennsylvania State University, October 2001.

Appendix

At an international meeting of Teen STAR held in Krakow, Poland, July 9-12, 2000, teachers from 17 countries were able to identify 22 program strengths. Among those related to the topic at hand were:

1) Students can be themselves, become more mature and self-directed

2) Teen STAR demands self-discipline, which is counter-cultural

3) Teen STAR moves girls from being victims of their hormones to being in control

4) Teen STAR encourages students to think ahead and to make decisions ahead of crisis

5) The program offers methods to reject peer as well as media pressure

6) Teen STAR enhances movement from middle to late adolescence, thereby enhancing students' level of ego development

7) Teen STAR affirms the youth's right to know about their own sexuality and helps them find answers (to their questions).

Response to: Undergirding Abstinence within a Sexalit Education Program
An Analysis of Outcome Data of the 1999-2001 Teen Star Program"
Alice B. Heinzen, M.A.
NFP Coordinator, Diocese of La Crosse, WI

We are at a turning point in the world of teen chastity programs. According to current research done by the National Campaign to Prevent Teen Pregnancy stopping teen sexual activity and promoting chaste behaviors in youth is a multi-faceted project. The underlying causes of sexual activity outside of marriage are numerous. Typically called risk factors, the short list of antecedents to premature sexual activity include community advantage or disadvantage, family structure, economic status, family-peer-partner attitudes and behaviors, academic success and the individual persona of the teens themselves. It is very important for all of us to understand that according to the "powers to be" in the secular research world these factors must be explored if we want to encourage more teens to save sex for marriage.

Those of us at this conference, who read this list, ask, "Why isn't a general understanding of human sexuality and fertility awareness part of this list?" Good question! Perhaps it is because those of us who work in the teen chastity field have not been able to convince those in the secular research world that the understanding the body and fertility has a great impact on chaste behaviors.

The report that I received, "Undergriding Abstinence Within A Sexuality Education Program" submitted by Dr. Hanna Klaus with Mary Nora Dennehy and Jean Turnbull presents the findings of the impact of fertility tracking and awareness on a teen's ability to stay chaste or return to chaste behaviors. This report on an abstinence-only program highlights that a basic understanding of the biological capacity to mother or father a new life is a very important factor that may reduce teen sexual risk taking. According to Dr. Klaus, "it seems that until youth can 'own' their fertility more than just intellectually they cannot integrate their sexuality and become more mature. Only after coming to terms with the fact that one is now biologically capable of becoming a mother or a father, can awareness of this capacity be integrated into choices about present behavior which are consistent with future goals."

I believe that Dr. Klaus' premise is correct—knowledge and experience in charting one's own fertility patterns may be a crucial element in empowering youth to withstand the sexual pressures. When a young person understands the physiological and affective impacts of cycling hormones in females or the consistency of hormone levels in the male, he or she is given a new control over his or her body and actions that are taken. This concrete knowledge of fertility may lead to more self-awareness and discipline, both of which are vital in maintaining or regaining chastity.

Those of us who work in the field of abstinence-only sexuality programs know what Dr. Klaus knows – when a young person understands who they are both physically and emotionally, they feel more in charge of their actions and that they tend to act in ways that protect their sexuality. Unfortunately, there is a group of researchers in the U.S. who do not believe as we do that abstinence-only programs are effective. In a recent report, Dr. Douglas Kirby, a renowned researcher in the field of teen sexuality states, "Very little rigorous evaluation of abstinence-only programs has been completed…none showed an overall positive effect on sexual behavior." (Kirby, 2001, 8). In the same report, Kirby goes on to relate that sex and HIV education programs and improved access to condoms and contraceptives are effective in limiting teen sexual activity and teen pregnancies. We know that abstinence-only programs are superior and do more to preserve the dignity and value of each young person. Yet, abstinent-only programs are not being recognized in the "greater world" of teen sexuality because they don't have peer reviewed research to back them up.

Chastity and abstinence-only educators count on well designed, rigorous research to bring credibility and reliability to their work. It is my hope that Dr. Klaus and her colleagues will use these preliminary results to generate a very rigorous evaluation of the impact of fertility awareness on teen sexual activity. It is my desire that well known leaders in our field, as Dr. Klaus is, will execute sound, research protocols on the correlation between fertility awareness and teen chastity, or work in concert with other chastity education leaders to prove the thesis that those who understand and respect God's design for human fertility are most likely to recognize sexual activity as a gift and act more maturely.

Abstinence-only programs like Teen Star have the potential to turn many persons back to holy and healthy sexual practices and increase the number of youth and young adults who will save sex for marriage. But, we must understand that in today's skeptical society, only peer reviewed, solid study and research is recognized and taken seriously. Thus, I urge both Dr. Klaus and all others who promote teen chastity to engage in rigorous, reliable studies.

Bibliography

Kirby, D. 2001. *Emerging Answers Research Findings on Programs To Reduce Teen Pregnancy (online)*. Washington, D.C. The National Campaign to Prevent Teen Pregnancy, 2002 [cited 15 June 2002]. Available from World Wide Web: (http://www.teenpregnancy.org/resource/data/pdf/emeranswsum.pdf)

Klaus, H. 2001. *Undergirding Abstinence Within A Sexuality Education Program* (online). Bethesda, MD. The Teen Star Program, 2002 [cited 21 October 2001]. Available from the World Wide Web: (http://www.teenstar-international.org/)

A Life History Study of Sexually Abstinent, Adolescent, African American Females

Kristin Haglund, Ph.D. R.N.
Asistant Professor, Marquette University

Nationally, 61% of youth have initiated sexual intercourse by the twelfth grade (CDC 1998). There is ample evidence that many of these youth experience adverse consequences of sexual activity. Each year there are approximately 1,000,000 teenage pregnancies in the U. S., most (75%) of which are unplanned. Additionally, 3,000,000 adolescents, or about 1 in 4 sexually experienced teens, contract sexually transmitted infections (STIs) annually (Ozer et al.1998). Some youth may also experience adverse psychological or spiritual consequences of sexual activity, such as guilt, shame or remorse, or adverse interpersonal consequences such as strained relationships with parents or harassment from peers.

In response to these problems, adults frequently have promoted the practice of sexual abstinence as an effective way to prevent the adverse consequences of sexual activity. However, too often abstinence interventions are designed and presented by adults without input from adolescents themselves. Efforts to encourage abstinence may be more successful if adolescents participated in the development of interventions by identifying areas in which they have knowledge and areas that they are lacking knowledge or have erroneous knowledge; identifying specific contemporary issues related to abstinence such as peer pressure, pressure from romantic partners or influence of popular media; and finally identifying ways to deliver the intervention so that the adolescent audience is engaged, interested and intrigued.

In addition to the lack of data about how adolescents describe abstinence, there is a lack of data about how adolescents actually experience abstinence. Few studies have focused on the factors that influence youth to be sexually abstinent although many have investigated factors that influence the initiation of sexual intercourse. Information from successfully abstinent youth regarding what factors help them and what factors make if difficult for them to maintain abstinence is critical to the development of effective, meaningful abstinence interventions. Thus the findings of this study represent first steps towards improving the efficacy of abstinence interventions by providing an adolescent-centered description of sexual abstinence and descriptive information about the contexts that support and inhibit sexual abstinence.

While sexuality is salient for male and female adolescents, this study included only female adolescents due to marked gender differences in the experience and consequences of adolescent sexuality. Adolescents receive mixed messages about sex that are gender linked. In general, possession and expression of sexual desire is considered to be normal in adolescent males. To many, it is natural and desirable for males to express their virility. Whereas female adolescents are often characterized as potential victims of the oversexed males who "must protect themselves against the desires of men outside of marriage" (Brooks-Gunn and Paikoff 1991, 534). Female sexuality is considered dangerous. Although this characterization of female sexuality is too limited, it does have a basis in reality. In many cases the consequences of sexual activity are more intense for females than males as adolescent females bear the brunt of the burdens of premature parenting and are at risk for serious long-term negative consequences from STIs such as pelvic inflammatory disease, HIV infection and cervical cancer. Thus given these distinctly different experiences, being sexually abstinent is also likely to be different for adolescent males and females.

Finally, this study included only African American females to refute the stereotype that African American females are hypersexual, seductive, and promiscuous. Negative stereotypes of African women developed long ago and were used to justify and perpetuate their exploitation, domination and oppression by white Europeans and later by white Americans during the time of slavery (Vaz 1995). Today, African American women are still characterized as hypersexual persons. In particular, there is a prominent view that most if not all African American adolescent females are sexually active and most of the girls will become teen mothers. This view is in fact false. The stories of these participants provided some evidence against these negative views.

Conceptual Perspective

The conceptual perspective of this study was the life span developmental approach. The life span approach is a family of perspectives that describe patterns of growth, stability and change in behavior throughout the life span (Smith and Baltes 1999). In the life span approach, human development is characterized as a life-long process that occurs in multidirections and within contexts, is modifiable, and is not the scientific province of one discipline but requires multidisciplinary perspectives.

Purpose

The purposes of this study were to: describe sexual abstinence from the perspective of female adolescents and to explore the contexts in which urban African American adolescent females were sexually abstinent.

Research Questions

1. How do adolescent, sexually abstinent African American females describe sexual abstinence?

2. What are the life experiences and relationships within and across contexts that influence adolescent, African American females to be sexually abstinent?

3. How do life experiences and relationships within and across contexts pose challenges to being sexual abstinent?

Methods

General Aims and Design

This study utilized a life history approach. The purpose of obtaining life histories was to gain an understanding of how past events and life long patterns influenced current behavior. This approach was consistent with the research goals of this study namely, to discover the processes, relationships and events within and across contexts that influenced young women to be sexually abstinent.

Sample

The sample was comprised of 14 sexually abstinent, African American females between the ages of 15.5 and 18 years with a mean age of

16.4. Participant recruitment closed after the 14th participant as the researcher stopped hearing substantially new themes and thematic saturation was reached. All of the participants described themselves as being African American except one who described herself as being an African Jamaican and who was an American resident. They all attended public high schools. Of the 14 participants, 12 were virgins. Eleven participants had had boyfriends and most had kissed boys, including three who said that they had "made out" with boys. Two participants had had sexual intercourse in the past, but not in the past year or longer.

Nine of the 14 participants reported regular church attendance. Thirteen belonged to Protestant Christian religious denominations and one said she had no religion. Eight participants had family incomes equal to or below the 2000 federal poverty level based on their family income and the number of persons in their household. One participant's family income level was above 133% of poverty and five participants' family income levels were above 185% of poverty. The participants lived in a variety of family arrangements including two parent, one parent, and guardian-headed households. All of the participants had siblings with the number ranging from one to seven. Three participants had siblings who had been a teen parent.

Procedures

Participants were recruited from a school-based health center located in a local high school, an adolescent pregnancy prevention program in which senior high school students taught abstinence to middle school students, and an adolescent primary care clinic. Parental and participant consents were obtained. Each participant completed two interviews on different days ranging from 40 minutes to 90 minutes. All of the participants completed both interviews.

Data Collection

Data were collected during two audio taped, semi-structured interviews. An interview guide was used to direct the life history interviews. The guide included a list of questions arranged in chronological order from birth to the present and covered the contexts of life that were expected to be central to the life of an adolescent including school, family, peers, activities, puberty and sexuality. Participants were also asked about how they described abstinence, their experiences of being abstinent, and barriers to abstinence that they had encountered.

Analysis

Each interview was transcribed. The researcher reviewed each transcription while listening to the audiotape to screen for errors and detect salient features of the conversation not included by the transcriptionist. The sets of interview transcripts for each participant were divided into narratives and then condensed to adequate paraphrases. Narratives included stories with boundaries, sections of conversation linked topically to an interview question, or descriptive information about people or repetitive past experiences. The narratives maintained meaning when removed from the surrounding text so that they could exist on their own (Riessman 1993; Denzin 1989). The adequate paraphrases were then constructed using a modified six-step procedure described by Polanyi (1989). This procedure required that the researcher carefully examine each narrative line by line and identify the elements that the participant most heavily emphasized. Participants indicated emphasis in a variety of ways such as speaking louder or in a different tone of voice, repeating phrases, or using descriptive words. The most emphasized portions of each narrative were extracted, paraphrased and put together to form the text of the adequate paraphrase. The completed paraphrases were then coded. The list of codes was generated from the data during the coding process. Ultimately the codes were organized into hierarchical categories in which the highest level labels were reasons for abstinence, definition of abstinence, activities, family, community, peers, problem behaviors, school, self, and sexuality.

Each set of transcripts was analyzed to generate an overview of each participant's life history. Then the data from all participants were analyzed as a whole. Reports for each code including all passages across participants coded with that label were printed. Passages in each report were compared to the others in the same report and to the researcher's overall impression of all of the interviews to identify common and unique themes. The researcher periodically referred back to the participants' actual words to facilitate the analysis and to ensure that that the findings were representative of the participants' experiences. The analysis revealed the participants' descriptions of abstinence and how abstinence was promoted or inhibited within various contexts.

Evaluation

Rigor was measured in terms of credibility, transferability, dependability and confirmability. Credibility is the faithful depiction of the participant's lived experiences, not the verification of a preconceived conception of those experiences (Sandelowski 1991). Credibility was achieved through prolonged engagement and observation, inclusion of multiple participants, and member checks. Transferability is the ability to transfer the conclusions to another setting or population. Transferability was minimally established by providing thick description, a range of participants' responses and experiences, and verbatim quotations so that a person using the research could judge the possibility of a transfer to an alternate population (Lincoln & Guba, 1985). Dependability and confirmability were achieved by using an audit trail. An audit trail was established with the documents of data collection and analysis, the fieldwork journal, participants' written feedback and final written report. Dependability means that a different researcher using the same data and analytical techniques and making the same methodological decisions would draw similar conclusions. Confirmability means that findings, interpretations and recommendations are supported by the data rather than reflecting researcher bias.

Protection of Human Subjects

IRB approvals for this study were obtained from the Institutional Review Board at the University of Wisconsin-Milwaukee and the Human Rights Review Board at Children's Hospital of Wisconsin. All names were changed and care was taken to not identify participants in the study and subsequent manuscripts.

Results

Participants' Descriptions of Sexual Abstinence

Being sexually abstinent is often described as a dichotomous experience; either one has had sex or not. However, abstinence was not so simplistically defined in these participants' descriptions. Abstinence was unanimously described as a behavior that one chose; lack of opportunity to have sex did not make one abstinent. Although across participants abstinence meant refraining from having sex, there was disagreement on which types of sexual behaviors were prohibited. The most conservative description of abstinence included refraining from all genital and breast contact, clothed or unclothed, as well as kissing. Others felt that unclothed breast contact or clothed genital contact were permissible for abstinent persons. Couples who engaged in penile-vaginal intercourse were unanimously considered not abstinent. Most, but not all participants, considered couples who engaged in oral-genital contact and anal intercourse to be not abstinent. The dissenters felt that couples who engaged in oral or anal intercourse without inserting the penis into the vagina were still abstinent. Finally, most felt that a person who had had vaginal intercourse could become abstinent again if they made a conscious commitment and refrained for at least one year. However, most were skeptical that a person could resist having sex again after sexual initiation.

Contextual Influences of Sexual Abstinence

Sexuality. The participants told many stories related to sexuality. The maturation processes they were undergoing, physical as well as emotional, spiritual and cognitive, had two functions in the development of their sexuality. First, the changes attracted attention from men and women that irrevocably identified "the once girls and soon to be women" were capable of intimacy and reproduction. Secondly, their new powers gained through maturation, such as observation, introspection, and perspective taking, provided them with the tools they needed to process their internal changes as well as the intense external influences. Each participant's sexuality was shaped by an array of influences including biology, physiology, interpersonal interactions and relationships, and their personal attitudes about sex, love and abstinence. The participants' cited a number of attitudes that supported their choice to be abstinence including a belief that they were waiting for Mr. Right, a commitment to high school graduation, a desire to set a positive example for younger youth, a dedication to a lifestyle that was consistent with their religious values, pride in their ethnicity and a desire to be a positive example of an African American person, and a sense of belonging and responsibility to their families.

The participants also experienced the most barriers to abstinence within the context of sexuality. They experienced frequent requests for sex from adolescent boys and sometimes from adult men. In general they ignored these requests although sometimes they thought it would be easier to give in rather than resist. Their boyfriends asked them for sex and broke up with them when they refused. Some teenage girls made fun of them for being virgins. Other sexually active girls told them that having sex was a pleasure that they should not be missing. Finally, they would lose friends when their formerly abstinent girlfriends became sexually active and stopped being friends with them. Thus it is remarkable that within a few short years and despite these barriers, the participants set abstinence as their standard and actively tried to live a life consistent with this standard.

Self. Most of the participants were involved in extracurricular activities which kept them busy and engaged so that they did not have time to think about having sex. All of the participants attended high school. Most were engaged in school and strived to achieve so that they could go on to college. Twelve of the 14 participants possessed one or more personal attributes that influenced them to be and to remain abstinent. Some felt that they were more mature than other teens their age, some valued being different from other teens and some said that they purposely avoided situations in which they could get in trouble. Being abstinent was one way they demonstrated their maturity, was something that made them different and was an effective way to avoid trouble.

Family. Family was an important part of the participants' lives and influenced them to be abstinent in a variety of ways. For most, their relationship with their mother was a central organizing feature of their lives. Even when their relationships with their mothers were strained, they continued to rely on her for economic and emotional support. The participants' admiration and respect for their mothers combined with a feeling that their mother was the most important person in their lives, led them to follow their mothers' rules even when they didn't like them. Following the rules contributed directly to abstinence as the rules were often designed to either prevent the participants from having boyfriends or were designed to prevent prolonged, unsupervised interactions with boys and boyfriends and to thereby prevent sexual activity. Mothers also influenced abstinence indirectly as they were the participants' role models of mature, independent and strong adult women. The participants wanted to be women like their mothers. Being abstinent was a way to show that they were mature and independent like their mothers.

Eleven of the 14 participants had men in their lives that they called father. Of these, seven participants described a close, consistent relationship with their fathers. The participants reported little discussion about sex, love or abstinence between father and daughter apart from the few instances when the fathers admonished the participants to stay away from boys and men altogether. However, as they valued their fathers' love and attention, maintaining abstinence may have been a way to preserve their special relationship with their fathers.

Siblings were each other's best friends. They protected, comforted and supported each other. Siblings influenced the participants to be abstinent by being each other's role models. Participants wanted to be like their siblings who had been abstinent throughout high school and did not want to like their siblings who had been teen parents. The participants with younger siblings were abstinent so that they would set a good example for these younger children.

The maternal grandmother had a special, vital role as the safety net for the family. Without her, many of the families in this study would have had severe hardships including homelessness, foster care and destitution. Thus the participants also saw their maternal grandmothers as role models of adult women who took care of their responsibilities. The participants' abstinence was again a way to demonstrate how they were becoming women like their mothers and grandmothers. In addition, grandmothers provided extra love and attention for the participants. This affection between participants and their grandmothers encouraged abstinence because the participants did not want to hurt or to disappoint their grandmothers and thereby jeopardize their relationship.

Religiosity. Eight participants cited religious beliefs as a reason for being abstinent. They were taught and believed that having sex outside of marriage was a sin. These participants were trying to live a Christian lifestyle, which included waiting until marriage to have sex. For these participants, faith was the mechanism through which religiosity influenced abstinence. They had faith in a God who they believed wanted them to be sexually abstinent, therefore their abstinence demonstrated their faith. Because they had faith, they regularly attended church services. Faith facilitated the transmission of the pastors' teachings about abstinence because they were physically present in church to hear them and because they believed in what their pastors were saying. They were active in social activities at their churches where they developed social relationships with other abstinent youth and with adults who expected them to be abstinent. These relationships further reinforced their abstinence.

Conclusions

Adolescents are often disparaged by adults who say that teenagers are self-centered and only concerned with the present that they cannot even conceive of future consequences. Teens are often considered to be incapable of making their own good choices because they are unable to resist peer pressure and blindly accept the messages of advertisers or celebrities. Because of the perceptions that adolescents are not good decision-makers, some adults advocate that sexuality information should be censored and restricted from them.

Contrary to these opinions, the participants in this study demonstrated a capacity for thoughtful, responsible decision-making. They had sexual information, although much of it came from their peers and was erroneous and even absurd. Nonetheless, the participants worked with the information that they had including some that encouraged sexual activity and some that supported abstinence, and made the choice to be sexually abstinent. Utilizing a variety of sophisticated cognitive skills such as perspective taking, projection and evaluation of future consequences, reflection, prayer, and cost-benefit analysis they were able to sort through the conflicting information, resist peer and media pressure and opt for abstinence. Their sincerity and commitment to a sometimes-difficult lifestyle set an example for other youth as well as for adults.

Thus adults, who are striving to guide youth into productive, healthy and happy adulthoods, should not be reticent to discuss sexuality with adolescents. In their search for an adult identity, sexuality is a salient issue. Accurate teaching about human reproductive anatomy and physiology, frank discussion about how sexual interactions occur, and explanations of how infections are transmitted and pregnancies are induced will prepare youth to combat the foolish things their friends say and help them to protect themselves now and in the future. In order for abstinence to be effective, youth must know how the consequences actually occur and then how abstinence works as a preventative measure. In addition to teaching the physical aspects of abstinence, talking to youth about aspects of healthy interpersonal relationships is also a critical. It is important to teach youth aspects of relationships such as how to be friends, how to be affectionate in safe ways, and how to negotiate and then respect personal boundaries in order for them to be prepared to maintain abstinence when faced with pressure from peers or romantic partners. Finally, youth should be made aware that maintaining abstinence takes work and commitment but is well worth the effort.

Bibliography

Brooks-Gunn, J., and Paikoff, R. 1991. "Promoting healthy behavior in adolescence: The case of sexuality and pregnancy." *Bulletin of the New York Academy of Medicine* 67 (6): 527-547.

CDC. 1998. "Trends in sexual risk behaviors among high school students —United States, 1991-1997." MMWR, 47 (36).

Denzin, N. 1989. *Interpretive Biography: Qualitative Research Methods*, Vol.17. Newbury Park: Sage Publications.

Lincoln, Y., and Guba, E. 1985. *Naturalistic Inquiry.* Beverly Hills: Sage Publications.

Ozer, E., Brindis, C., Millstein, S., Knopf, D., and Irwin, C. 1998. *America's Adolescents: Are They Healthy?* San Francisco, CA: University of California, San Francisco, National Adolescent Health Information Center.

Polanyi, L. 1989. *Telling the American Story. A Structural and Cultural Analysis of Conversational Storytelling.* Cambridge: The MIT Press.

Riessman, C. 1993. *Narrative Analysis: Qualitative Research Methods*, Vol. 30. Newbury Park: Sage Publications.

Sandelowski, M. 1991. "Telling stories: Narrative approaches in qualitative research." *Image* 23: 161-166.

Smith, J., and Baltes, P. 1999. "Life-span perspectives on development." In M. Bornstein & M. Lamb's (Eds.) *Developmental Psychology.* Mahwah, NJ: Lawrence Erlbaum Associates, Publishers, 47-72.

Vaz, K. 1995. Black Women in America. Thousand Oaks, CA: Sage Publications.

Comparison of Ecological Breastfeeding with Lactation Amenorrhea Method (LAM)

Sheila Kippley

Couple to Couple League, International

God's Plan for Mother and Baby

I am grateful for the opportunity to speak about breastfeeding. A couple who uses breastfeeding to space their babies is using Natural Family Planning (NFP). I commend the organizers of this conference for wanting to examine the contribution breastfeeding has played in NFP. Because this is a faith and science conference, I'd like to present some faith-based thoughts about breastfeeding and then offer the scientific aspects of breastfeeding with respect to natural infertility.

Breastfeeding and Church Teaching

Does the Catholic Church have any teaching on breastfeeding? Fr. William Virtue asked this same question in the early 1990s, and his search culminated in the publication of his book, *Mother and Infant*. Fr. Virtue states that "the testimony of the Magisterium and moral experts confirms that it has been the constant teaching of the Church that there is a serious obligation of maternal nursing" (Virtue 1995, 278). That is so strange to our ears that I want to repeat Fr. Virtue's statement. "The testimony of the Magisterium and moral experts confirms that it has been the constant teaching of the Church that there is a serious obligation of maternal nursing." We asked Fr. Virtue to clarify what he meant by serious obligation. By "serious," he doesn't mean "mortal sin serious," but he does mean serious and not just trivial.

Is there papal teaching on this subject?

According to Fr. Virtue, popes Gregory the Great, Benedict XIV and several saints taught the moral obligation for a mother to nurse her baby (Virtue 1995, 272). The teachings of two recent popes are better known. In 1941 Pius XII taught that the mother's influence and her education of the soul and body of her infant begin at the cradle. Thus Pius XII urged all mothers to breastfeed their babies, if at all possible (Yzermans 1961, 44).

In May 1995, John Paul II promoted the immunological, nutritional, and emotional benefits of breastfeeding. "This natural activity benefits the child and helps to create the closeness and maternal bonding so necessary for healthy child development" (John Paul II 1995, 14). The present pope encouraged mothers "to breastfeed for 4-6 months from birth and to continue this practice, supplemented by other appropriate foods, up to the second year of life or beyond" (John Paul II 1995, 15). "No one," he says, "can substitute for the mother in this natural activity" (John Paul II 1995, 15).

Catholic Church Documents

When the Church speaks of Natural Family Planning in such encyclicals as *The Gospel of Life* and *Humanae vitae*, such teaching applies also to breastfeeding. In both encyclicals, we are told to follow God's plan through His biological laws.

In *The Gospel of Life*, John Paul II writes as follows:

"There is a plan of God for life which must be respected" (no. 22).

"We are subject ...to [the] biological laws" (no. 42).

"We are told to "respect the biological laws inscribed in our person" (no. 97).

In *Humanae vitae*, Paul VI tells us to obey the natural law (no. 11), to consider the biological processes first (no. 10), and to observe those laws inscribed on our very nature by the Most High God if we are to be happy (no. 31)!

Breastfeeding is God's biological law

Breastfeeding is essential for life. There are only two voluntary acts between two persons that are necessary for the continuation or survival of the human race: the marital act between husband and wife and the breastfeeding act between mother and child.

Breastfeeding is a continuation of the care the child received from his mother during pregnancy. The baby has merely switched positions. In Scripture we are reminded of this continuity of care in 2 Macabees 7:27 when a mother tells her son, "I carried you nine months in my womb and nursed you for three years." There are three conditions present during pregnancy as well as during the breastfeeding:

1) The exclusive nourishment provided by the mother's body to her baby during pregnancy is continued after birth as the mother's body continues to provide exclusive nourishment again through breastfeeding.

2) The baby continues to receive that much needed touch and close physical contact by the mother through breastfeeding that the baby received from his mother during pregnancy.

3) During both pregnancy and breastfeeding, the mother usually receives many months of amenorrhea. Nature intends the typical mother to receive more months of amenorrhea through breastfeeding than through pregnancy.

Natural child spacing

In Scripture there is a hint of natural child spacing. In Hosea 1:8 a mother weans her child first and then she conceives and bears a son.

In *Humanae vitae*, I am reminded of breastfeeding when I read: "God has wisely arranged the natural laws and times of fertility so that successive births are naturally spaced (no. 11).

Natural Child Spacing and the Research

In the 1960s as a young Catholic mother I was very interested in breastfeeding infertility. The Catholic obstetrician I saw for my first pregnancy said that no matter how I nursed my baby I would have a return of menstruation by 3 months. I nursed frequently day and night, and, like he said, I did have a return of menstruation by 3 months postpartum. I saw a different Catholic obstetrician with our second baby; this doctor promoted the temperature method. However knowing I wanted to nurse my baby, he gave me the exclusive breastfeeding rule. I was told to only breastfeed, not to offer the baby even water, and to call him when menstruation returned. Menstruation returned a year after childbirth.

Why the difference between the two babies? I nursed both babies frequently day and night. I had attended La Leche League meetings prior to and after the births of our first two babies. I knew what kind of nursing was required to keep up an ample milk supply.

I searched for any scientific evidence to determine the validity of the statement that breastfeeding spaces babies. As I looked into the research and into the changes of my mothering practices with our second baby, I began to realize that mothering practices do directly affect the amount of nursing that occurs at the breast.

The research papers that I found, although dated from the 1930s to the 1970s, are not much different from the conclusions of current breastfeeding research that we have today (pre-seventies research is listed in the first editions of *Breastfeeding and Natural Child Spacing* published by Harper & Row in 1974 and Penguin in 1975). The research up through the 1960s focused on two main points:

1) suckling by the baby can inhibit the ovarian cycle of the mother after childbirth and

2) early supplementation causes an early return of fertility for the nursing mother.

I would like to compare a few old and new studies. In 1967 scientists stated the importance of suckling that is "applied periodically and at short intervals" for improved lactation (Grosvenor 1967, 453). Today Dr. William Taylor concludes that the frequent number of suckling sessions per day and a short spacing between each nursing session is what counts for the continuance of postpartum amenorrhea (Taylor 1999, 308).

In 1943, Dr. Paul Topkins concluded that during "the amenorrheic period of lactation, ovulation does not occur" (Topkins 1943, 57). In 1954, Dr. Thomas McKeown studied over 900 nursing mothers. In this study no mother conceived while exclusively breastfeeding and before they had their first period (McKeown 1954, 826). Today the Lactational Amenorrhea Method (LAM) stresses the importance of lactational amenorrhea and of exclusive breastfeeding in preventing conception (Consensus 1988, 1204).

In 1968, the year of *Humanae vitae*, Dr. T. J. Cronin concluded that "provided full breastfeeding is in progress and menstruation has not returned, ovulation does not happen before the end of the 10th postpartum week" (Cronin 1968, 424). This 1968 knowledge fits in well with the Bellagio Consensus of 1988 which states that any vaginal bleeding can be ignored for the first 56 days or first 8 weeks postpartum in determining the mother's fertility if the mother is exclusively breastfeeding (Consensus 1988, 1204).

One doctor stands out above all the rest because of the duration of his research on breastfeeding and natural child spacing from the 1950s to the 1970s. Dr. Otto Schaefer researched breastfeeding conception rates among the Canadian Eskimos for over twenty years and showed how breastfeeding can impact a nation as well as the individual family. He concluded that the small size of the traditional Eskimo family was due to prolonged lactation. From the mid-1950s to the mid-1960s, he recorded a 50% increase in the birthrate among the Eskimos due to the exposure of baby bottles at the trading posts. "The shorter the distance [to the trading posts], the more frequently they had children" (Schaefer 1971, 15-16). The older Eskimo women, 30-50 years of age, had conceived their babies 20-30 months after childbirth due to prolonged lactation, while the younger women under 30 year of age, were conceiving 2-4 months after childbirth due to bottlefeeding and shortened lactation (Schaefer/Hildes 1971, 6).

My husband and I also decided to do some research. An extensive survey was placed in the first edition of our self-published book, *Breastfeeding and Natural Child Spacing,* beginning in June 1970. In our analysis, the first sign of bleeding or spotting, no matter how early, was counted as a first period. If amenorrhea was reestablished, we recorded amenorrhea only by the first bleeding. For statistical analysis, any response of 1.0 to 1.9 was recorded as 1.0. We excluded any nursing mother who had an unusually long amenorrhea, such as 40 months or longer. In other words, our analysis was quite conservative.

The determination of what constituted ecological breastfeeding was set by six criteria. These six criteria are very similar to the Seven Standards for breastfeeding infertility that the Couple to Couple League promotes today:

No pacifiers used
No bottles used
No solids or liquids for first 5 months
No feeding schedule other than baby's

Presence of night feedings
Presence of lying-down nursing for naps and night feedings

In 1971 we had 112 nursing experiences from 72 American mothers. Of those, 29 nursing experiences from 22 mothers followed the ecological breastfeeding or natural mothering program. Those mothers averaged 14.6 months of amenorrhea (Kippley 1972).

After collecting surveys for 15 years, we had over 1500 breastfeeding experiences. A data analysis computer program was developed and a student nurse was hired to work the summer of 1985 to enter the data into the computer. The surveys were not pre-selected. We stopped inputting the data when the additional surveys showed no differences. Of 286 surveys recorded, there were 98 nursing experiences that qualified as ecological breastfeeding using the same Six Criteria as in the first study. These ecologically breastfeeding American mothers averaged 14.5 months of amenorrhea—essentially the same as the 14.6 months in the 1971 study (Kippley 1989, 107-116). We concluded that there is no question that American couples can and do experience extended breastfeeding amenorrhea and natural baby spacing provided they do the right kind of breastfeeding.

We tried to discover if there was any single one of the six criteria for ecological breastfeeding that by itself showed an even greater duration of amenorrhea, but we found none (Kippley 1989, 111). What we have discovered over the years is that the elimination of any one of the practices usually brings an earlier return of fertility.

Ecological breastfeeding with its frequent and unrestricted suckling of the baby at the breast is nature's way of spacing babies. God in His wisdom provides many benefits to the nursing mother and her baby, one being natural child spacing.

Today we talk about the Seven Standards to describe the type of breastfeeding that provides frequent and unrestricted suckling and thus a natural extended amenorrhea for the mother (Kippley 1999, 2). Each of the Seven Standards is important in its contribution to natural infertility. These Seven Standards are as follows:

1. Do exclusive breastfeeding for the first six months of life; do not use other liquids and solids.

2. Pacify your baby at your breasts.

3. Do not use bottles and pacifiers.

4. Sleep with your baby for night feedings.
5. Sleep with your baby for a daily-nap feeding.
6. Nurse frequently day and night, and avoid schedules.
7. Avoid any practice that restricts nursing or separates you from your baby.

What is the natural norm?

Here we are looking to the norm of nature and not to the sociological norm or the norm that society expects. Frequent and unrestricted nursing is the norm. Extended breastfeeding is nature's norm. Extended amenorrhea is nature's norm. To have a period return by three months postpartum is the exception, not the norm, by nature's standards.

The effects of various types of breastfeeding upon fertility

Our first consideration is cultural or restricted nursing. This is the type of nursing that is common in the United States. Some like to call it *restricted* nursing, since they hope that eventually cultural nursing will be similar to ecological breastfeeding.

Restricted nursing occurs when the mother uses pacifiers, bottles, early supplementation, babysitters, and strict schedules. This type of nursing has been studied extensively. Let's look at a study that is the best in the sense that these mothers took their breastfeeding a little more seriously than in the other studies. These mothers nursed for a longer period of time, and this study had the highest rate of amenorrhea at 6 months postpartum. Of the 485 mothers who nursed their babies for at least one month after birth, 38% were in amenorrhea at 3 months postpartum, but only 9% of the original 485 nursing mothers were in amenorrhea at 6 months postpartum. Further, of the 485 who nursed for at least one month after childbirth, only 111 mothers or 23% were still nursing at 6 months (Salber 1966, 351). In most studies involving restricted nursing, most weaning occurs during the first few months after childbirth.

Our second consideration is exclusive breastfeeding. Exclusive breastfeeding is where the mother offers *only* breast milk to her baby. The American Academy of Pediatrics (1997), UNICEF (1993, 1999) and the WHO (IFBAN 2001) all encourage mothers today to nurse exclusively for the first 6 months of life.

In 1988 a group of international experts met in Bellagio, Italy to review all the scientific literature about breastfeeding infertility. The conclusion of this group about breastfeeding infertility has become known as the Bellagio Consensus: a woman who is fully or near fully breastfeeding during the first six months postpartum has a "more than 98% protection from pregnancy" if she remains in amenorrhea. In determining amenorrhea, any vaginal bleeding during the first 56 days can be ignored (Consensus 1988, 1204).

The exclusive breastfeeding rule today is often called the Lactational Amenorrhea Method (LAM). The best study involving the exclusive breastfeeding rule occurred at Santiago, Chile and was reported in 1992. I say "best" because the number of those mothers still in amenorrhea at 6 months was greatest in this lactation amenorrhea study. Of the 422 nursing mothers studied, 56% were still in amenorrhea at 6 months postpartum (Perez 1992, 970). During these six months postpartum, this study showed a 99.6% non-pregnancy rate for these exclusively breastfeeding mothers before menstruation occurred (Perez 1992, 968).

More current studies dealing with the LAM have changed the definition of amenorrhea so that a certain amount of bleeding is allowed (Labbok 1997, 329). The definition of exclusive breastfeeding has changed to allow an infant to take a slight amount of supplement to breast milk each week, the supplement increasing slightly at each month postpartum (Labbok 1997, 329).

In these current studies of the LAM two rules were also added to the exclusive breastfeeding rule to encourage frequent nursing among the mothers and thus achieve results closer to the results of ecological breastfeeding. These rules are:

1) Night feedings should be given and
2) "Intervals between breastfeed should not exceed 4 hours during the day, and 6 hours at night" (Labbok 1997, 328).

Basically, current studies of the LAM often stress the importance of night feedings and "no long intervals between breastfeeding" (Hight-Laukaran 1997, 343; Peterson 2000, 225). These additional changes have produced mixed results. In 1997, 62% and, in 2000, 53% of the nursing mothers using the LAM were in amenorrhea at six months postpartum (Labbok 1997, 332; Peterson 2000, 225).

In my work over the last 35 years, I have always been aware that an early return of menstruation is common among mothers who do only exclusively breastfeeding. I used to tell parents to picture an "ecological breastfeeding" pie. There are seven pieces to the pie and exclusive breastfeeding is only one piece of the pie. Too frequently exclusively breastfeeding mothers are disappointed to experience menstruation at 3 or 4 months postpartum. It is for this reason that those who promote breastfeeding and the LAM or the exclusively breastfeeding rule for amenorrhea emphasize the importance of frequent suckling day and night so that more mothers will enjoy six months of amenorrhea with a 98-99% natural infertility rate.

For example, UNICEF says, "If a baby sucks very frequently at the breast (whenever the baby wants to, including at night), then the return of the mother's periods will be delayed for much longer." Again this organization says, "Breastfeeding gives a mother 98% protection against pregnancy for six months after giving birth—if her baby breastfeeds frequently, day and night, if the baby is not regularly given other food and drink, and if the mother's periods have not returned" (1993). Thus certain researchers and promoters of the exclusive breastfeeding rule are describing baby-care practices that approximate ecological breastfeeding in some respects.

The third consideration is ecological breastfeeding. Ecological breastfeeding is described by the Seven Standards. In our late 1980s study of the mothers who were involved in ecological breastfeeding, 93% were in amenorrhea when their babies were six months old. That compares with 9% with restricted nursing and 56% with exclusive breastfeeding. At 12 months, 56% of those ecologically breastfeeding were in amenorrhea. That's the same as the LAM at 6 months. At 18 months, 34% of the mothers doing ecological breastfeeding were still in amenorrhea (Kippley 1989, 111).

Let's conclude with a practical example. Imagine that you have a hundred mothers who want to experience the natural amenorrhea and infertility that God has built into breastfeeding, what will you teach them?

If they are taught a restricted nursing pattern, only 9% will still be in amenorrhea at six months postpartum.

If they are taught the Lactation Amenorrhea Method or the exclusive breastfeeding rule, about 56% will be in amenorrhea at six months.

If they are taught ecological breastfeeding, 93% will be in amenorrhea at six months and will receive the natural infertility rate of 99% during the first six months postpartum. Furthermore, if they continue with ecological breastfeeding, they will have their first period, on the average, around 14½ months postpartum, and a third will still be in amenorrhea at 18 months.

The only type of breastfeeding associated with extended natural infertility or natural child spacing is ecological breastfeeding. The best answer is to teach ecological breastfeeding to all new mothers-to-be so they will be fully informed.

Bibliography

American Academy of Pediatrics. 1997. "Breastfeeding and the Use of Human Milk." (Policy Statement). *Pediatrics* 100: 1035-1039.

Consensus Statement. 1988. "Breastfeeding as a Family Planning Method." *The Lancet* 332: 1204-1205.

Cronin, T. J. 1968. "Influence of Lactation Upon Ovulation." *The Lancet* Aug. 24, 1968; 2 (7565): 422-424.

Grosvenor, C. E., Mena, F., and Schaefgen, D. A. 1967. "Effect of Nonsuckling Interval and Duration of Suckling on the Suckling-Induced Fall in Pituitary Prolactin Concentration in the Rat." *Endocrinology* 81: 449-453.

IBFAN. 2001. "WHO's Global Strategy for Infant and Child Feeding Settles Duration of Exclusive Breastfeeding." *IBFAB Info* (The International Baby Food Action Network newsletter) 3:2.

John Paul II. 1995. "Breastfeeding: Science and Society." Pontificiae Academiae Scientiarum Documenta 28, (May 11-13). Or "Breastfeeding Protects Against Disease and Creates Bond of Love." *L'Osservatore Romano* (May 24, 1995).

Kippley, S. 1999. *Breastfeeding and Natural Child Spacing*. Cincinnati, Ohio: The Couple to Couple League Int.

Kippley, S. K. and J. F. 1972. "The Relationship Between Breastfeeding and Amenorrhea: Report of a Survey." *Journal of the Nurses Association of the American College of Obstetricians and Gynecologists* 1: 15-21.

Kippley, S. K. and Kippley, J. F. 1989. "The Spacing of Babies with Ecological Breastfeeding." *International Review.* 13:107-116.

McKeown, T., and Gibson, J. R. 1954. "A Note on Menstruation and Conception During Lactation." *Journal of Obstetrics and Gynaecology* 61: 824-826.

Perez, A., Labbok, M. H., and Queenan, J. T. 1992. "Clinical Study of the Lactational Amenorrhea Method for Family Planning." *The Lancet* 339: 968-970.

Salber, E. J., Feinleib, M., and MacMahon, B. 1966 "The Duration of Postpartum Amenorrhea." *American Journal of Epidemiology* 82: 347-358.

Schaefer, Otto. 1971. "When the Eskimo Comes to Town." *Nutrition Today* 6: 8-16.

Schaefer, O., and Hildes, J. A. 1971. "Health of Igloolik Eskimos With Urbanization." Circumpolar Health Symposium presentation, Oulu, Finland.

Taylor, W., Vazquez-Geffroy, M., Samuels, S. J., and Taylor, D. M. 1999. "Continuously Recorded Suckling Behaviour and Its Effect on Lactational Amenorrhoea." *Journal of Biosocial Science* 31: 289-310.

Topkins, P. 1943. "The Histologic Appearance of the Endometrium during Lactation Amenorrhea and Its Relationship to Ovarian Function." *American Journal of Obstetrics and Gynecology* 45: 48-58.

UNICEF. 1993. "Breastfeeding." *Facts for Life.*

UNICEF. 1999. "Breastfeeding: Foundation for a Healthy Future."

Virtue, Rev. William D. 1995. *Mother and Infant.* Rome: Pontifica Studiorum Universitas.

Yzermans, V. A. 1961. *The Major Addresses of Pope Pius XII: Vol. 1 Selected Addresses.* St. Paul: North Central Publishing.

Arguments against Contraception
Do They Make Sense to the General Public? Importance of ethics, religion and "natural morality" in choice of family planning methods

Rafael Mikolajczyk, M.D.
Department of Gynecology and Obstetrics
Otto-von-Guericke University of Magdeburg,
Magdeburg, Germany

Joseph Stanford, M.D.
Department of Family and Preventive Medicine,
University of Utah, Salt Lake City, USA

Introduction

Contraception is almost universally accepted in modern societies and the majority of Catholics in developed Western countries do not adhere to their Church's doctrine prohibiting its use. The discrepancy between doctrine and behavior of Catholics is not fully understood. Whereas some dissenting Catholic theologians emphasize the proper decision of the ordinary person's conscience for contraception, researchers point to a low importance of ethical or religious issues in the choices most couples make about family planning. Previous studies have focused on behavior of different religious denominations or the stated importance of moral or religious issues for family planning choices. We undertook a detailed examination of the perceptions of patients about arguments against the use of contraception

Based on the phenomenology of the human body three arguments to reject contraception can be developed, all related to "natural morality" or intuition about the inherent nature of the human body:

1. The totality of marital love, including the complete mutual giving of the marital act, which may be compromised by excluding fertility through contraception,

2. The importance of the fertility cycle as an inherent language of the human body, which may be compromised or eliminated by the use of some contraceptive methods,

3. The integrity of the human body that may be endangered by some contraceptive procedures.

In order to understand the interactions between ethics, religion and "natural morality" we studied the agreement with the above arguments translated into statements related to particular contraceptive methods and compared this "natural morality" with the formal importance of religion across different cultures.

Methodology

A self-administered comprehensive written questionnaire was distributed to 860 post-partum women, 239 responded in Berlin and 249 in Cracow (overall response rate 57%). The questionnaire included demographic, religion, and religious commitment items, a detailed examination of history and choices of family planning and reasons for choice, and statements to address "natural morality" arguments. Berlin was chosen to represent predominantly secular society and Cracow for a heavily religious society (Catholic).

Results

Similar education and employment levels and different marital status and confession were found in both study groups. (See Table 1)

There was a higher religious commitment in Catholics in Cracow, compared to Catholics and Protestants in Berlin. (See Figure 1)

A considerable proportion of respondents in both groups agreed with the statements based

Tab. 1. Socio-demographic characteristics of the studied groups (%)

		Berlin	Cracow
Religion	Protestant	14,9	-
	Catholic	7,9	98,8
	Others	5,1	-
	No religion	72,1	1,2
Marital Status	married	55,0	92,2
	not married	45,0	7,8
Educational Level	primary	10,0	5,8
	«medium»	65,0	67,4
	university	25,0	28,8
Employment	no job, housewife	14,6	19,7
	jobless	3,8	3,1
	medical	12,2	10,3
	in training	11,7	7,6
	others	57,2	59,2

Arguments against Contraception

Fig. 1. Comparison of religious commitment (mean on scale including importance of faith in personal life, commitment to the own religious community and attendance of services)

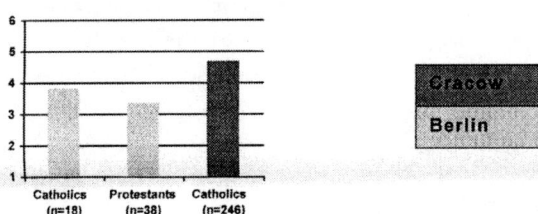

on "natural morality," there was a little difference between groups despite the strongly differing religious background. (See Table 2) There was a major difference in the declared importance of ethical or religious issues in the choice of family planning methods (much higher importance in Cracow) and there was agreement in the level of importance of ethical or religious issues in the choice of family planning methods and the "natural morality" statements in Cracow,

Tab. 2. Assessment of "natural morality" statements (% of respondents who agreed or strongly agreed)

	Berlin	Cracow
I would consider sterilization to be an injury to myself.	60,9	79,5
To me, using the pill would mean consciously rejecting my own fertility.	41,6	60,4
Using chemicals [for birth control] would manipulate my body.	44,8	49,1
I think using a condom would be an assault on the wholeness of the sexual union	21,0	33,3
Using the pill disturbs the innate functions of my body.	31,1	45,9
The use of contraception keeps fertility out of the complete giving of sexual intercourse.	12,6	25,3
Contraception opposes fertility.	31,0	35,9
Using the pill denies you the opportunity to consciously reckon with [your] fertility.	20,7	37,8
Contraception prevents using the fertility cycle as a means for mutual understanding in the marriage or partnership.	8,1	36,7

whereas in Berlin there was a dissociation between them both. A comprehensive agreement on "natural morality" (held by about 20% of respondents in Cracow) was associated with a high use of Natural Family Planning (NFP). (See Figure 2)

Conclusion

We conclude that while many people accept contraception within their cultural context, they still hold at least some beliefs that are consistent with the rejection of contraception, and probably also the acceptance of NFP.

Fig. 2. Comparison of declared importance of ethics/religion with the agreement on "natural morality" statements in bot groups (mean % of respondents who agreed or strongly agreed)

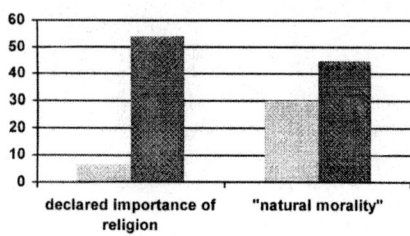
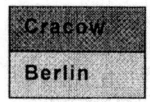

We further conclude that there is an association between a more comprehensive agreement with arguments against contraception and the use of NFP. Whether this latter association is because the experience of NFP use alters beliefs or because a stronger set of beliefs leads to NFP use cannot be ascertained from our study.

However many questions remain, among them the following:

1. Would Catholics (and others) who hold these beliefs while still using contraception, actually decide to reject contraception given the appropriate circumstances, or are there other beliefs that we did not measure that would override in favor of contraception?

2. Could helping people understand these reasons for rejecting contraception lead to more effective promotion of NFP?

Introduction to the Ovarian Monitor and Applications for Assessment Practice and Research

Leonard F. Blackwell, Ph.D.
Institute of Fundamental Sciences-Chemistry, Massey University, Palmerston North, New Zealand and Health & Fertility Foundation, Palmerston North

Introduction to the Ovarian Monitor

In this presentation I want to address some important questions relating to the Ovarian Monitor and its use in NFP and elsewhere. I propose to do this under four main headings. Any one considering using the Ovarian Monitor for the first time will no doubt have a number of questions among which would be; (1) "What is the Monitor?" (2) "How does it work?" (3) "How well does it work"? and (4) "What can be done with it?" At a meeting such as this the last question is likely to become "How is the Monitor to be used in natural family planning (NFP)?"

It is important to understand in this presentation that I am talking about two distinct things. The most important is what I call the knowledge base. This consists of the total knowledge on the human menstrual cycle in all its aspects obtained by any analytical system. This knowledge represents the hard facts about fertility and is independent of methodology. The second aspect is the device we call the Ovarian Monitor (or Monitor for short) which is designed to make the knowledge available to whoever wishes to use it. Without such a device the knowledge is of academic interest.

When speaking about the Monitor around the world I have noticed that the usual response is that the Monitor is in need of further development and hence the knowledge I present obtained by the Monitor must also be in need of further development and can be ignored. This is a great pity and a loss especially to NFP. As I hope to show the information produced by the Monitor is the equal of most laboratory methods and the understanding of the cycle it has given will stand no matter what other device or devices may be produced.

(1) What is the Monitor?

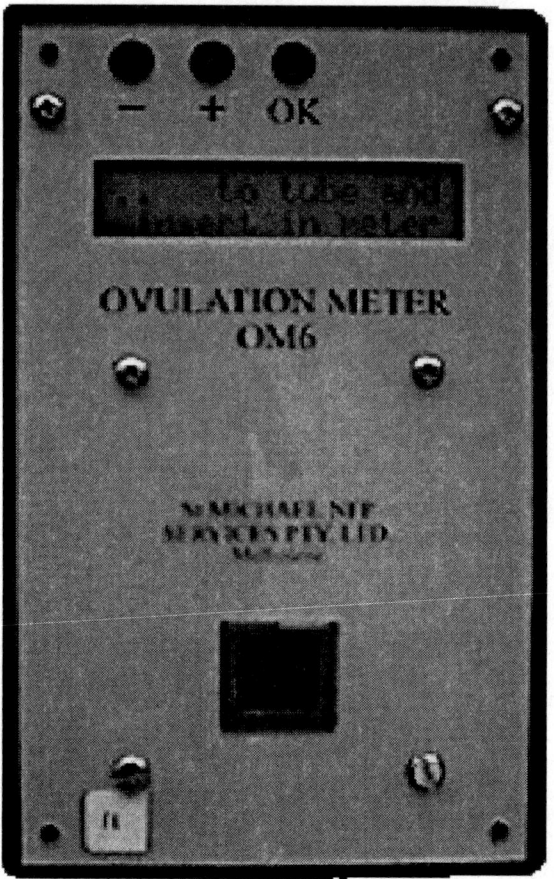

Figure 1. Picture of Ovarian Monitor Mark 6.

The Monitor is a system consisting of a simple colorimeter (Figure 1) and an assay tube (see Figure 2 for example) which measures a rise in estrone glucuronide (E1G) above a woman's early follicular phase baseline as a marker for the beginning of the potentially fertile phase (Blackwell and Brown 1992). A second assay tube is used to measure the rise in pregnanediol glucuronide (PdG) to equal or exceed a threshold value as the end marker (Blackwell et al. 1998). The Monitor has been developed over the past nineteen years and at each stage it has been validated against reference assays or by similarly rigid criteria (Brown et al. 1988; Brown, et al. 1989; Brown et al. 1968; Brown et al. 1978; Barrett and Brown, 1970).

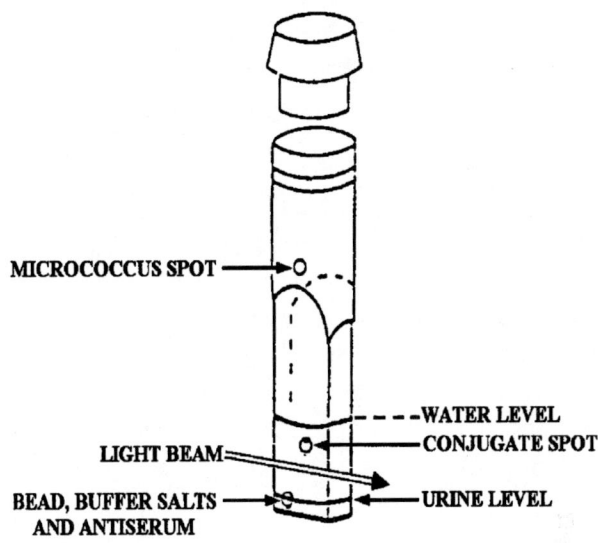

Figure 2. Schematic of a typical ovarian monitor assay tube.

A typical hormonal profile obtained by a woman at home during the World Health Organization (WHO) sponsored study of the Ovarian Monitor is shown in Figure 3. This display is from a program we have written called OMAssist which allows daily graphical display of Monitor and mucus data as the cycle unfolds. This cycle is the second from participant 002F2 in the WHO-sponsored trial of the Monitor and shows the E1G, PdG and mucus data for the entire cycle of 25 days. Since all women have a more or less constant baseline of urinary estrogens resulting from peripheral conversion of adrenal androgens the contribution to the total output from the emerging follicle is seen as a rise above the early follicular phase baseline (Brown et al. 1989). The E1G rise occurs on day 9 and the mucus change from the basic infertile pattern (BIP) occurs on day 8. The peak E1G excretion rate occurs on day 13 which is the same day as the mucus peak symptom

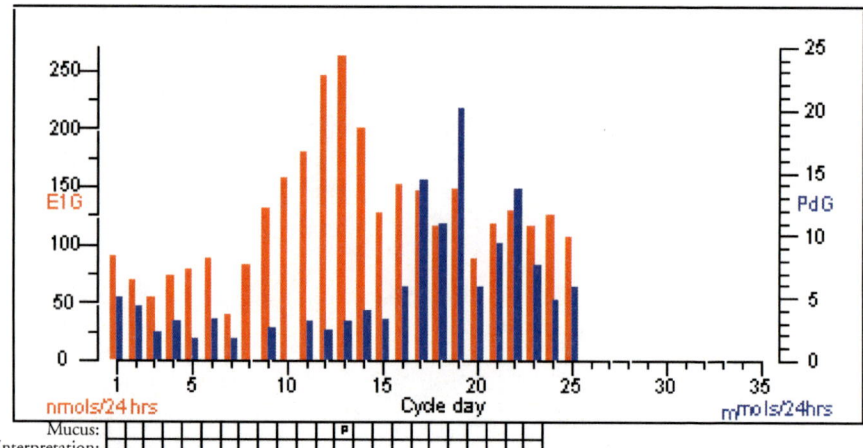

Figure 3. Computer display of the daily E1G and PdG from a full ovulatory cycle obtained during a study of the ovarian monitor. E1G in red and PdG in blue.

(defined as last day of fertile symptoms). Thus the hormones give about 6 days warning of ovulation (which occurs in the 36 hours following the E1G peak day) and the mucus symptom gives 7 days warning. The PdG threshold is exceeded on day 17 which means that the last day of the fertile window is day 16 or about 1 day earlier than given by the mucus peak + 3 days. The luteal phase is 12 days and the PdG

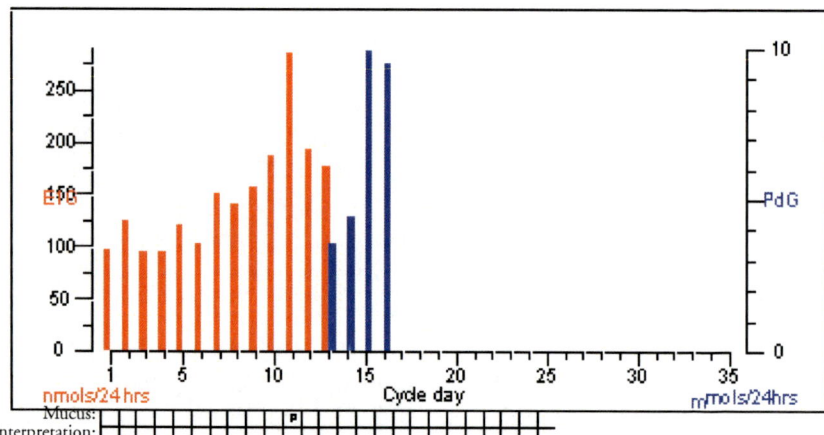

Figure 4. Computer display of use of the monitor in the third and subsequent cycles during the study of the ovarian monitor. The E1G data were measured until the mid-cycle.

values exceed 10 μmol/24 h on at least one day showing that this is a normal ovulatory cycle.

Figure 4 shows the fifth cycle from participant 023B. In this cycle the woman collected the E1G data only, until the rise and fall was observed and then did the PdG tests only, until the threshold was exceeded. This represents a more likely usage of the Monitor and could be simplified further by integrating it with the mucus symptom. In this example the E1G rise occurred on day 7 while the woman was still bleeding and the E1G peak excretion day was 5 days later on day 11 again giving about 6 days warning of oncoming ovulation. The mucus peak symptom also occurred on day 11 but there were only two prior mucus days (days 10 and 11). The end of fertility was indicated by the PdG measurements on day 14, or the same day as indicated by the mucus peak symptom. In this cycle the daily E1G measurements would give more security in the follicular phase.

These two examples serve to illustrate the basic use of the Monitor

1. When the E1G levels rise above the previous baseline a dominant follicle is present.

2. When the E1G levels having risen, then fall, ovulation may be due and this is the most fertile day.

3. The fate of the follicle is indicated by the PdG levels. Once the PdG level has equalled or exceeded the threshold value the fertile period is already finished.

(2) How does the Monitor work?

This has been published elsewhere (Brown et al. 1988, 1989) hence I will merely summarise the underlying theory. The assay depends on the fact that steroid glucuronide conjugates of the enzyme lysozyme are extensively inhibited by the appropriate anti-steroid glucuronide antibody. This is a result of steric blocking of access to the active site of the enzyme. Three dimensional structures of a lysozyme conjugate and the anti-E1G/E1G-lysozyme conjugate show that the large bacterial substrate for lysozyme (*M. luteus*) cannot approach the active site. As a result the enzyme in the immune complex is essentially inactive. Hence a simple measurement of the lytic activity gives a direct measure of the hormone concentration and no separation steps are needed. All of the reagents can therefore be freeze dried into a single assay tube (Figure 2).

The Ovarian Monitor (Mark VI) unit is controlled by an automatic timer and a microchip, and consists of a cell holder housed in an electronically heated block with a 40°C thermostat, a 650 nm light source (light emitting diode) and a detector (see Figure 1). Because separate assay tubes are required for the E1G and PdG assays and the timing requirements for the two assays are different, the Ovarian Monitor has been designed to differentiate electronically between the two tubes which are essentially the same except for their antibody specificity and the nature of their steroid glucuronide conjugates. In each tube, the *M. lysodeikticus* spot is freeze dried near the top of the tube, the conjugate spot approximately midway, and the buffer salts and the antibody spot together with a small glass mixing bead at the bottom. Upon the assay being initiated the instructions are highlighted step-by-step, on the liquid crystal display according to the identity of the assay tube.

The timed urine sample requires the collection of a single void (collected over 3-10 hours) into a jug calibrated in hours (150 mL hr^{-1}). The sample is then diluted by eye with tap water up to the nearest quarter hour according to the collection time. The timed urine speci-

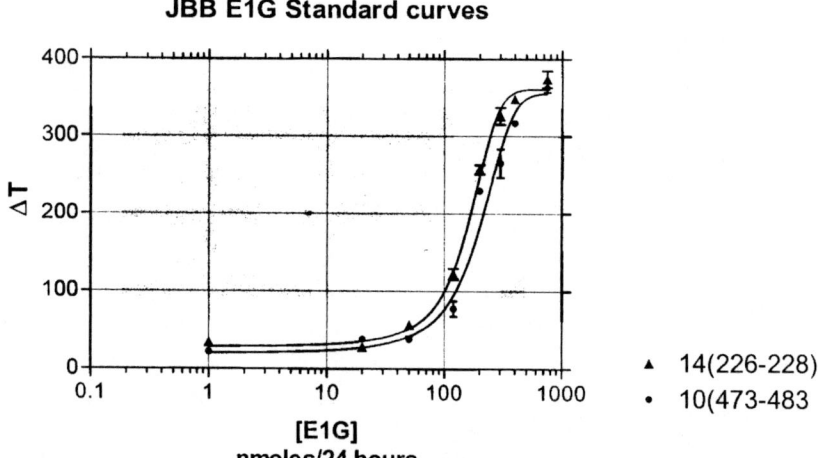

Figure 5. A diagram of a standard curve for E1G relating the monitor response to the concentration of E1G.

men (50 µL) is added to the bottom of the appropriate assay tube (Figure 2) where it reacts with the antibody partially neutralising it (step 1,). Then water is added to wash the second (conjugate) spot into the solution where it reacts with the remaining antibody (step 2,). The amount of free enzyme and hence the enzyme activity is determined by the amount of E1G in the urine sample. The substrate is then shaken up and the rate of lysis (or clearing) determined by the transmission change over 20 minutes for an E1G measurement and 5 minues for a PdG measurement (step 3,). A typical standard curve is shown in Figure 5 for E1G. The women merely record the ΔT value each day as their record of the hormonal pattern but this can always be converted into appropriate units by reference to the standard curve.

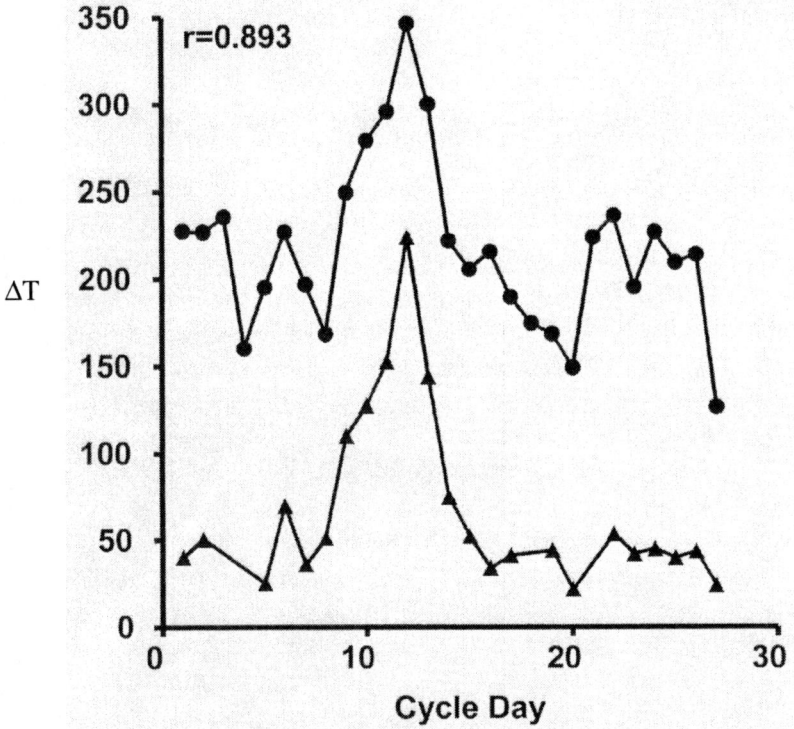

Figure 6. Comparison of a monitor E1G cycle with the correpsonding data obtained by a reference radioimmunoassay (RIA).
Monitor data in filled circles and RIA data in filled triangles.

(3) How Well does the Monitor Work?

This was established by us to our satisfaction in Melbourne by 1988 but the World Health Organisation wished to check this during a multicentre study involving 60 regularly ovulating women in three centers one of which was Palmerston North. For the first two cycles the women performed daily assays of E1G and PdG (as in Figure 3) hence this gave the ideal opportunity for an independent assessment of the Monitor. We have carried out our own analysis of these data which I will now summarise. Figures 6-8 show the correlation of two of our cycles for which the Monitor E1G and PdG data and the radioimmunoassay (RIA) E1G and PdG data were obtained in London.

The patterns were clearly similar as shown visually and by the good correlation coefficient between the two methods. Although a good correlation was obtained the presence of the urine blank effect we see with the Monitor assay for E1G is clearly demonstrated. This shows up in the fact that the absolute E1G values of the urines are clearly higher for the Monitor but the important fact to notice is that the *patterns* are the same. This is visually apparent and is reflected in the

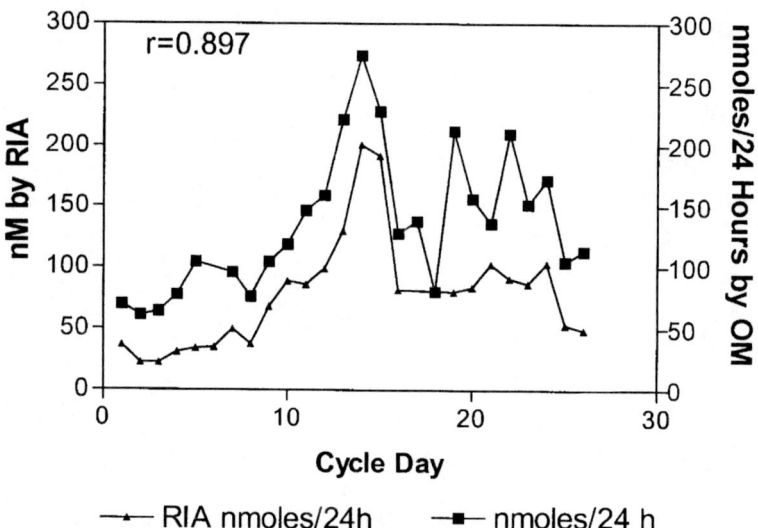

Figure 7. A similar comparison showing a cycle with a lower urine blank effect for the monitor data. E1G data in filled squares, RIA data in filled triangles.

correlation coefficient of 0.893. All of the individual cycles were correlated in this way (Blackwell et al. 2003).

Figure 7 shows similar daily data for cycle 020K1 from the WHO study. Again the profile obtained with the Ovarian Monitor parallels cloesly that obtained by the reference radioimmunoassay at least until the mid-cycle E1G peak (and ovulation) has occurred. The absolute values for the E1G excretion rates are again higher for the Ovarian Monitor data but the difference is less than shown in Figure 6. Despite the existence of the urine blank the woman can still access all of the important infomation contained in the hormone measurements. The same information about the interchange between the ovary and the hypothalamus/pituitary is contained in both sets of data. It should be remembered that the important message-bearing data comes from the period from menses to the time of the fall in E1G levels in mid cycle. The luteal phase E1G data do not appear to contain vital information and are therefore irrelevant. This emphasizes the necessity of considering each woman as an indivdual and underlines the importance of using a rise from a woman's own baseline estrogen values as the marker for the beginning of the potentially fertile period (Blackwell and Brown, 1992).

The PdG correlations are excellent. The PdG data for cycle 020K1 from the WHO study (Figure 8) shows that although there are differences in the absolute values the patterns correlate to a very high degree. The PdG rises occur on the same day and exceed the threshold value of 6.3 µmol/24 hours on day 19 giving the last day of the fertile window as day 18. In conjunction with the first E1G rise on day 11 (Figure 7) a fertile window of 8 days can be calculated for this cycle with 5 days warning of ovulation. The luteal phase was 12 days and the PdG levels by both the Ovarian Monitor and the RIA showed that the cycle was a normal ovulatory one. Similar results were obtained for the 20 cycles which were analysed independently in London. A correlation of the entire data set showed that for PdG the Monitor is as good as comparable laboratory methods (Blackwell et al. 2003).

For the entire study we found that the differences between the first E1G rise day and the day of first mucus change from the BIP were almost normally distributed but for about 4% of the cycles the mucus symptom was too early by 6-17 days (Figure 9).

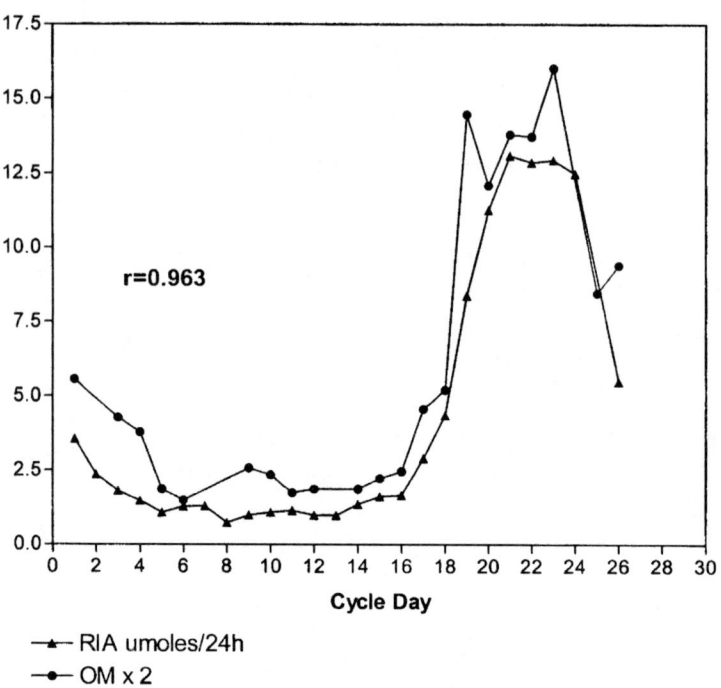

Figure 8. A comparison of the PdG data for the monitor (circles) and a reference PdG RIA (triangles).

Similarly for the E1G peak days and the mucus peak days with the mucus peak day occuring about 0.5 day later on average (Figure 10). The distribution of the days when the PdG excretion rate equalled or exceeded the threshold value was plotted against the day of the E1G peak is shown in Figure 11. The mean for reaching the threshold was 3.2 days after the E1G peak and the beginning of post-ovulatory infertility was on average 1.5 days earlier than for the peak mucus symptom.

The important conclusions which can be drawn from all of the comparisons are;

1. The Monitor is an accurate measure of urinary E1G and PdG patterns.

2. There is a high degree of correlation with independent reference assays.

3. The Monitor values are as informative as laboratory assays and are as reliable as markers of the fertile phase such as LH-5 to LH + 2. In fact they are more reliable since they monitor the ovarian activity as it occurs and do not assume a regular pattern of activity.

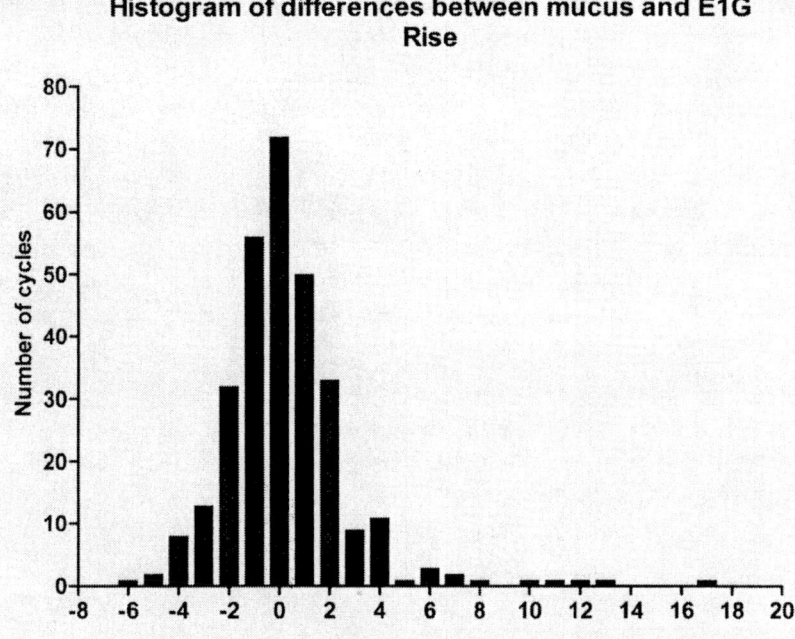

Figure 9. A histogram showing the differences between the beginning of fertility as indicated by the mucus and the first rise in E1G.

4. Neither of these markers is significantly superior to the mucus symptom for a population of regular ovulating, spacing women. For them, the hormonal markers are of little advantage apart from the increased certainty they give and the extra freedom for intercourse provided by the use of the PdG threshold which occurs on average 1-2 days earlier than the mucus peak day + 3 days.

5. The Monitor involves more labour, motivation and cost.

6. The women see little advantage over NFP but learn a lot about their fertility.

7. Given the complexity of the continuum of possible hormonal patterns the hope for a simple YES-NO answer for NFP is unlikely to be realised.

Uses of the Monitor in NFP

Despite the above comments the Monitor has an important part to play in NFP and we have gained much experience over the past 12 years about its role. Since we had already validated the Monitor against

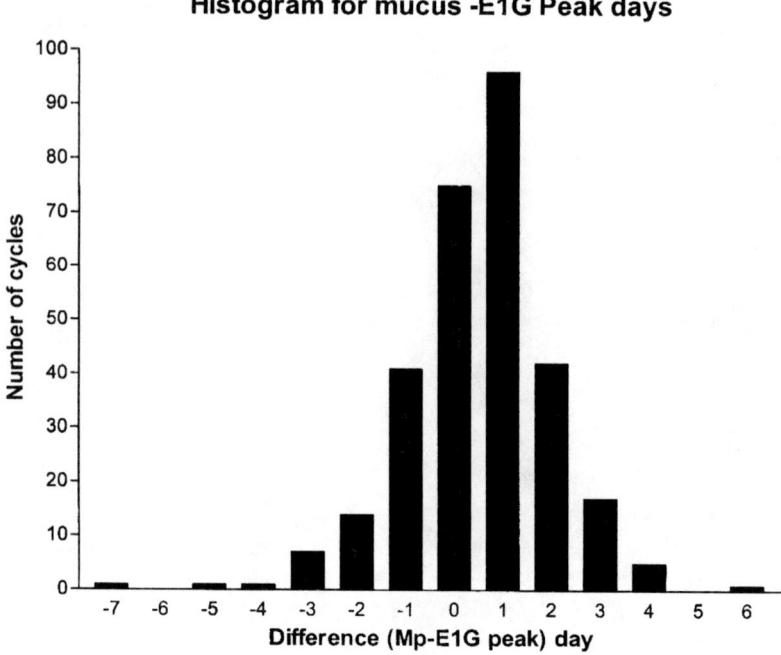

Figure 10. A histogram showing the difference between the mucus peak days and the E1G peak days.

our own reference assays and extensively correlated the results with the cervical mucus and BBT by 1988 (Brown et al. 1988) we continued to expand our use of the Monitor in fertility and infertility mainly in Australia while we waited for the WHO to repeat our validations. A summary of the place of the Monitor in NFP can now be given as a result of this effort.

The first woman to use the Monitor to sort out a difficult mucus symptom presented us with her superb results in December 1989. Including the hormone assays done before then and since with the Monitor we have accumulated approximately 1 million estrogen plus preganediol assays which represents about 50,000 cycles or 4000 woman years of experience. Approximately 50% of this use has been in NFP and 50% in infertility studies. One to two pregnancies have been encountered per year during this experience. Most of these have arisen from the use of the early follicular phase combined with a 5-6 day sperm survival or from intercourse without checking the estrogen

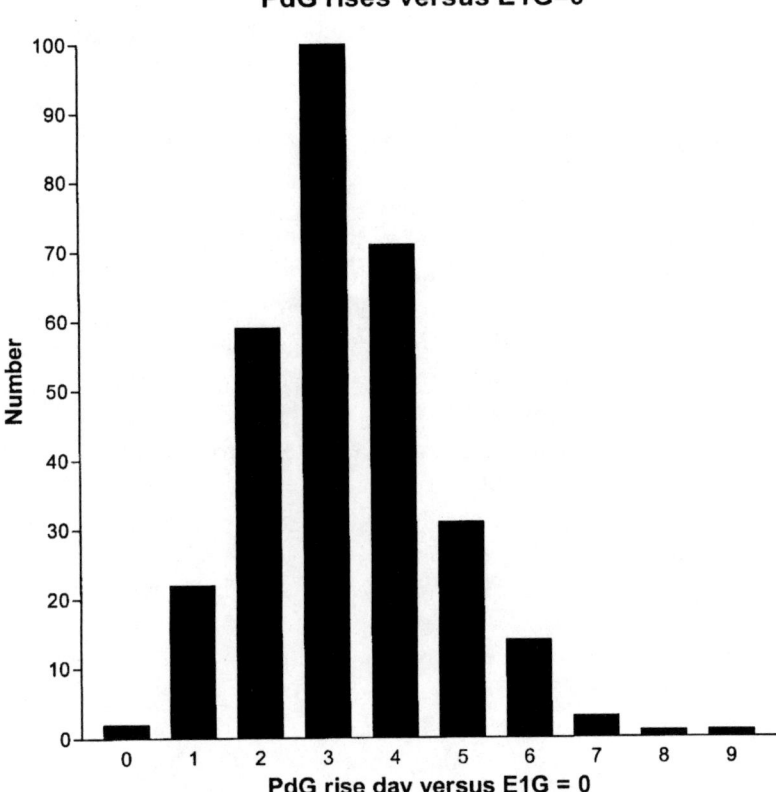

Figure 11. A histogram showing the rise in PdG excretion rate to equal or exceed the threshold value relative to the day of the E1G peak as zero.

values in a cycle when ovulation occurred early. There have been no pregnancies from use of the PdG rise marker.

The complete range of ovarian activity from no follicular activity at all, through follicular activity with attempted ovulation, follicular activity with ovulation and deficient luteal phase, full ovulation and finally enhanced ovulation has been defined. This range is called the continuum (J.B. Brown, personal communication). The associated symptoms have been defined, the fertility of each phase determined and which phase can be followed by a fertile ovulation without an intervening bleed has been determined. All of this is basic knowledge for the further perfection of NFP and has been discussed in the accompanying paper.

Monitor users in NFP fall into two categories; family spacers who are usually regular ovulators and family limiters and those who have irregular or difficult cycles. For the spacing group NFP works well so in the main they see no advantage in the Monitor. There is occasional use in this group to sort out problems and as a learning exercise. The main user group has been the women without completely regular cycles. Almost half of these have had a previous unplanned pregnancy with NFP and they want no more. This group is a forgotten group in NFP. They find the Monitor useful in the informed application of NFP and they form a highly motivated group to whom the extra labour involved in using the Monitor is regarded as being amply repaid. They use the mucus (Ovulation Method Billings) and the Monitor. It is important to appreciate that they need access to supervisors and educational backup to help them with their interpretation of the results just as NFP clients normally do.

The efforts of this group has led to the formulation of rules for use of the Monitor in all different situations encountered in NFP. For example breast feeding women, women with perimenopausal cycles, for timimg of intercourse, for gonadotrophin therapy, for difficult mucus symptoms and so on. One important conclusion which underpins all of the rules is that one should not expect stereotyped patterns. Also when monitoring ovarian activity do not ignore the hormone values no matter what you expect; they are very unlikely to be wrong.

As an example of the use of the Monitor, I will now conclude this talk with a brief discussion of the rules for breast feeding women established in Melbourne, Australia. To begin with the women establish their own E1G baseline by daily testing for 7 days. This will be recorded in nmoles per 24 hours but the woman will be given a baseline value applicable to her for each batch of tubes. The results are then interpreted as follows. If the E1G level remains below the baseline and the PdG level remains below the cut-off then those days are infertile. On the other hand if the E1G levels are above the baseline and the PdG levels are low these days must be regarded as fertile.

The frequency of testing depends on the time post-partum. If the woman is in the period 0-6 months post-partum she checks her E1G levels twice per week. If the E1G levels are below the baseline then the days are infertile. If however the E1G level is above her personal baseline or there is a change from the basic infertile pattern the woman notifies her contact person for advice. If she has a history of early return to fertility before 6 months she checks her urine samples three times per week from 0-2 months. From 6 months to weaning the E1G level is checked every third day and from 9 months to weaning the E1G test is done every second day.

The action to be taken following a rise in E1G is as follows. There may of course be a fertile ovulation. In this case the E1G levels will continue to rise for 3-7 days and then fall. After the E1G fall the PdG test is done to see whether it rises above the cut-off value in which case no further testing is necessary until the menstrual bleed. In the case of sporadic rises the following protocol is adopted. If there is a rise for only one day with no change in the BIP then the day of elevated E1G is unavailable for intercourse. However, if the E1G level returns to baseline with no change in the BIP then infertility continues.

If the E1G rises and remains above the baseline for 2 days or more the woman continues testing and looks for a fall in the E1G level. Then she tests for PdG. If the PdG level rises above the cut-off then (luteal phase) infertility has resumed. If however, the PdG values remain low for 2 or 3 days then E1G is tested for a further 3 days. If the E1G value returns below the baseline then the woman is back to a state of low fertility.

Similar protocols are available for other applications of the Monitor in NFP and some of these will be discussed in the afternoon session. Other experience has been published (Thornton et al. 1990; Brown et al. 1991; Cavero, 1995; Nolan 1996).

Acknowledgements

I wish to acknowledge the collaboration over many years of my friend and colleague Professor James Brown, Dr Meg Smith, Joanne Holmes, Gill Barker all of Melbourne and my students from Palmerston North, Yinqiu Wu, Mark Smales, Delwyn Cooke, Bryce Cummock, Zhao Zhang, Treena Blythe and Simone Flight.

Disclaimer

The material presented in this paper is based largely on information and data generously provided by Professor James Brown from Melbourne, Australia. In particular, the concept of the continuum is entirely from Professor Brown. Many of the figures are adapted from the Melbourne work with permission and from the WHO sponsored study of the Ovarian

Monitor. The opinions expressed are the authors but result from many hours of discussion with Professor Brown. Any errors of interpretation are my responsibility.

Bibliography

Barrett, S.A. and Brown J.B. 1970. "An evaluation of the method of Cox for the rapid analysis of pregnanediol in urine by gas liquid chromatography." *Journal of Endocrinology* 47: 471-480.

Blackwell, L.F. and Brown J.B. 1992. "Application of time-series analysis for the recognition of increases in urinary estrogens as markers for the beginning of the potentially fertile period." *Steroids* 57: 554-562.

Blackwell L.F., Brown, J.B., and Cooke, D. 1998. "Definition of the potentially-fertile period from urinary steroid excretion rates. Part II. A threshold value for pregnanediol glucuronide as a marker for the end of the potentially-fertile period in the human menstrual cycle." *Steroids* 63: 5-13.

Blackwell, L.F., Brown, J.B., Vigil, P., Gross, B.A., Sufi, S., and d'Arcangues, C. 2003. "Hormonal monitoring of ovarian activity using the Ovarian Monitor, Part I. Validation of home and laboratory results obtained during ovulatory cycles by comparison with radioimmunoassay." *Steroids* 68: 465-476.

Brown, J.B., MacLeod, S.C., Macnaughtan, C., Smith, M.A., and Smyth, B. 1968. "A rapid mrthod for measuring oestrogens in urine using a semi-automatic extractor." *Journal of Endocrinology* 42: 5-15.

Brown, J.B., Harrisson, P., and Smith, M.A. 1978. " Oestrogen and pregnanediol excretion throughout childhood, menarche and first ovulation." *Journal of Biosocial Science* Supplement 5: 43-62.

Brown, J.B., Blackwell, L.F., Cox, R.I., Holmes, J.M., and Smith, M.A. 1988. "Chemical and homogeneous enzyme immunoassay methods for the measurement of oestrogens and pregnanediol and their glucuronides in urine." *Progress in Biological and Clinical Research* 285: 119-138.

Brown, J.B., Blackwell, L.F., Homes, J. M., and Smyth, K. 1989. "New assays for identifying the fertile period." *Internation Journal of Obstetrics and Gynecology* Supplement 1: 111-122.

Brown, J.B., Holmes, J.M., and Barker, G. 1991. "Use of the home ovarian monitor in pregnancy avoidance." *American Journal of Obstetrics and Gynecology* Supplement 185: 2008-2011.

Cavero, C. 1995. "Using the ovarian monitor as an adjunct to natural family planning." *Journal of Nurse Midwifery* 40: 269-276.

Nolan, M.T. 1996. "Using the ovarian monitor as an adjunct to natural family planning." (Letter) *Journal of Nurse Midwifery* 41: 55.

Thornton, S.J., Pepperell, R.J., and Brown, J.B. 1990. "Home monitoring of gonadotrophin ovulation induction using the Ovarian Monitor." *Fertility and Sterility* 54: 1076-1081.

Eavesdropping on the Ovary
Hormonal Correlates of Fertility in the Human Menstrual Cycle

Leonard F. Blackwell, Ph.D.
Institute of Fundamental Sciences, Department of Chemistry, Massey University, Palmerston North, New Zealand

The central problem of fertility detection is to identify the fertile window in a menstrual cycle. This is a variable period of days surrounding ovulation when an act of coitus may result in a pregnancy. Since the position of the day of ovulation is usually quite variable even within cycles from the same woman the fertile window will vary from cycle to cycle and from woman to woman. The length of the fertile window will also vary from cycle to cycle and from woman to woman. It is generally agreed that the ovum only survives for 8-12 hours after ovulation but sperm survival in the female genital tract extends the fertile window by an amount determined by the sperm survival time. This is generally believed to average about 3 days however we have documented pregnancies which seem to require a rare survival time of up to 6 or 7 days. Hence the maximum length of the fertile window can be 7-8 days.

For Natural Family Planning (NFP) it is essential to identify the beginning of the fertile window and its end irrespective of where these days actually occur in a cycle. Also of importance is to identify the most fertile day of the cycle for those couples who wish to achieve a pregnancy. The aim of this paper is to show how these crucial days can be identified by home hormonal monitoring of the cycle. It is still a challenge being adressed by Professor Fehring of Marquette University and others, of integrating these measurements with a woman's signs and symptoms to identify the best time for testing. In this way the best information can be obtained with a minimum of testing. To understand this it is first necessary to review the basic physiology of the human menstrual cycle.

The Menstrual Cycle

The menstrual cycle is controlled by a coordinated flow of chemical information between the ovary and the pituitary gland as shown in Figure 1. The major chemicals which carry the information are the pituitary hormones, follicle stimulating hormone (FSH) and luteinising hormone (LH) which carry information to the ovary and the ovarian hormones, estradiol (E2) and progesterone (P) which signal ovarian responses to the pituitary. This orchestrated chemical com-

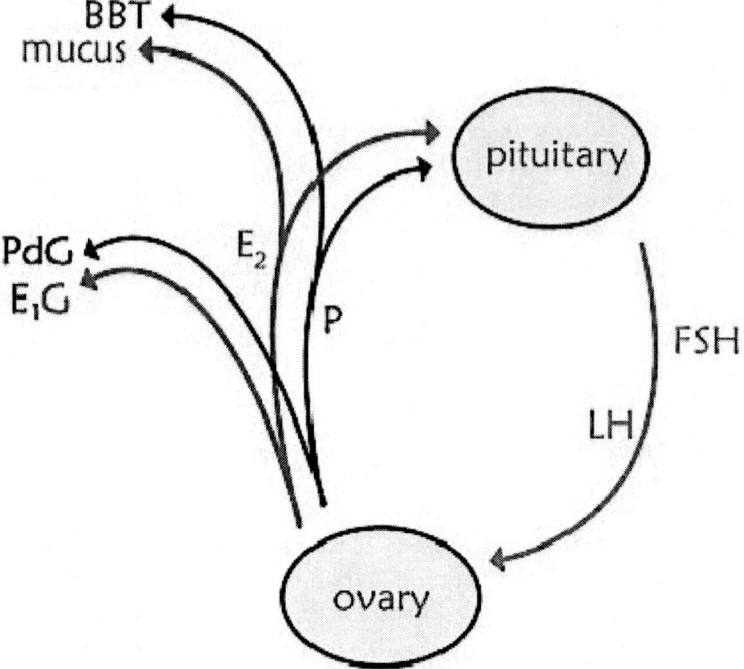

Schematic diagram of pituitary-ovary communication

Figure 1. Schematic diagram of pituitary-ovarian communication.

munication flow provides a means for eavesdropping non-invasively on the ovary to ascertain the state of follicular and corpus luteum development (and hence the state of fertility) at any time throughout the menstrual cycle. All of the available or forseeable methods of detecting and predicting fertility depend on access to a procedure which detects one or more of the signals shown in Figure 1. For example, Natural Family Planning (NFP) methods operate by monitoring the cervical mucus which is related to the E2 and P levels and the basal body temperature which is associated with progesterone. The Ovarian Monitor measures the urinary metabolites estrone glucuronide (E1G) and pregnanediol glucuronide (PdG) which are derived from estradiol (E2) and progesterone (P) respectively, in timed urine samples. It should be noted that no matter which method is being used the meaning of the underlying information remains the same. Hence the first part of this discussion is common to all NFP methods and needs to be understood clearly.

Fertility is critically dependent on a number of key events in this information exchange which I will call milestones. These occur in an ordered time sequence throughout the cycle for normal cycle behaviour to be observed. Of course fertility depends as well on the lifetime of spermatozoa in the female genital tract which depends on the quality of the cervical mucus. The first milestone (Figure 2) involves a gradual increase in the circulating levels of FSH (along with a basal level of luteinising hormone (LH)) until the threshold of the most sensitive follicles in the ovary is exceeded (Brown 1978). Figure 3 shows a plot of the number of follicles visible on an ovary throughout a menstrual

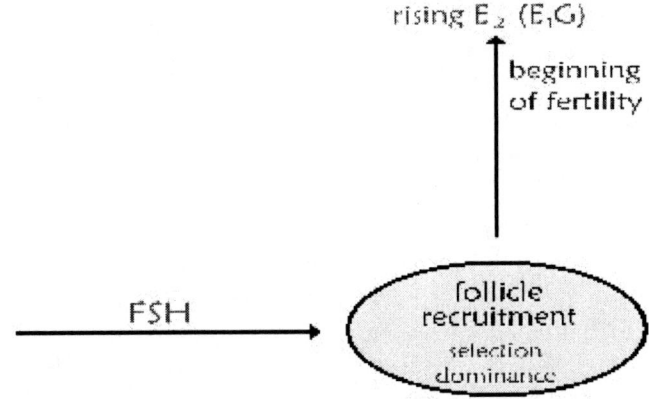

First Milestone

Figure 2. First milestone - follicle recruitment and dominance.

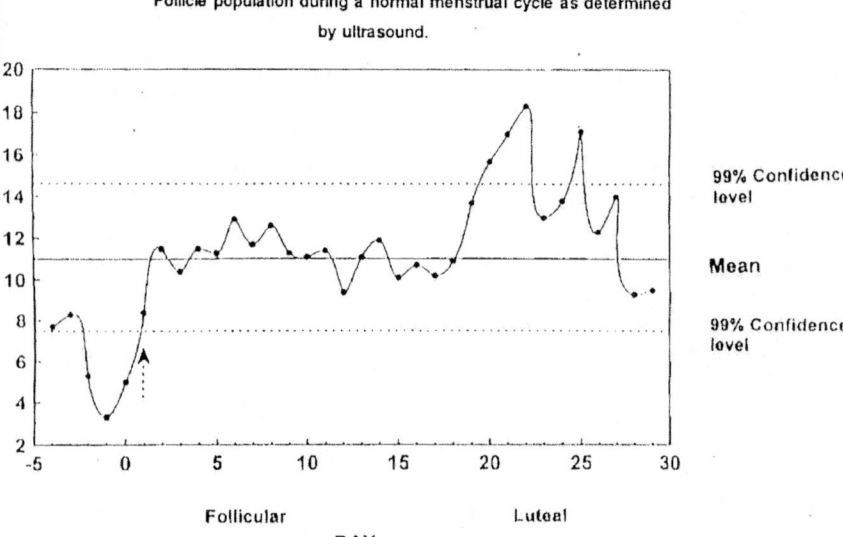

Note only one of these continues to ovulation.

Figure 3. Ultrasound determination of recruited cohort of follicles (from Nayudu and Gore).

cycle. At the beginning of the cycle the average number follicles increases to around 11 and this number is maintained throughout the cycle. However only one of these will ovulate. The emergence of the dominant follicle can be monitored in ultrasound, (Gore et al. 1997) as shown (Figure 4), being clearly identifiable among the other follicles all of which become atretic. The dominant (ovulatory) follicle is shown in black and the arrow indicates the time of ovulation. The diameter of the dominant follicle grows at an average rate of 2.4± 0.7 mm per day (Doody et al. 1987) and this is one of the characteristics of a normal cycle. McNatty (1983) showed some years ago that there was a corrrelation between the diameter of a healthy follicle and the maximum number of granulosa cells which it contained. Hence the rate of increase in diameter of an average dominant follicle can be replotted in terms of the maximum number of garanulosa cells (Figure 4). If the output of estradiol from each granulosa cell is approximately the same the linear growth in diameter of the dominant follicle will be reflected by a non-linear increase in estradiol or its metabolites. This is the basis of the familiar logarithmic increase in the output of urinary estrogens during a menstrual cycle.

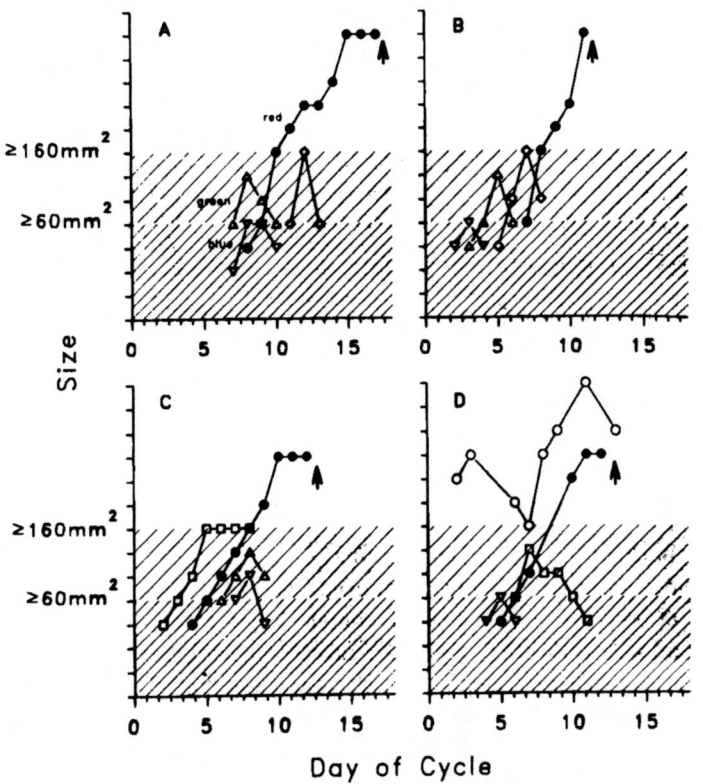

Figure 4. Ultrasound determination of domnant follicle emerging from the recruited cohort. From Nayudu and Gore)

Thus, the ovary signals the fact that a dominant follicle is present by sending out increasing concentrations of E2. This rising level of E2 above the previous baseline levels tells the hypothalamus/pituitary system to decrease the output of FSH (via the negative feedback system) to prevent development of more than one dominant follicle.

The second milestone (Figure 5) occurs if the estradiol level continues its (logarithmic) rise for a sufficient period of time (usually

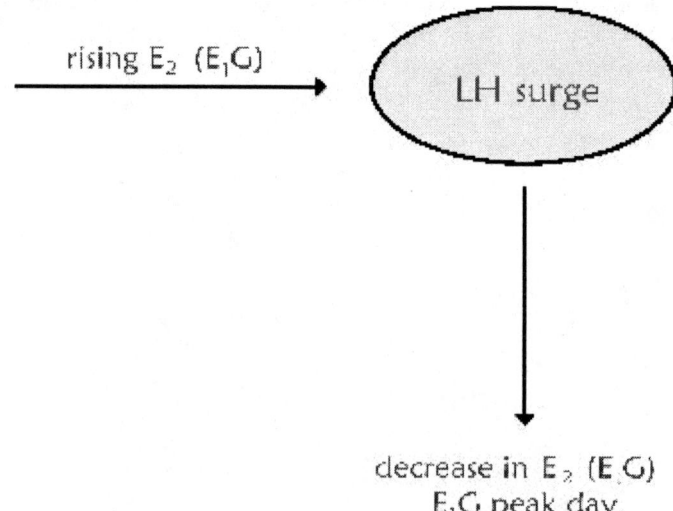

Figure 5. Second milestone - the LH surge.

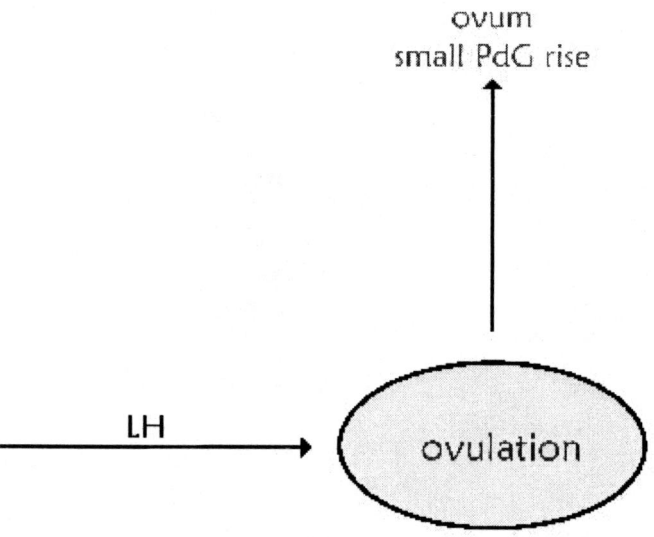

Figure 6. The third milestone – ovulation.

Eavesdropping on the Ovary

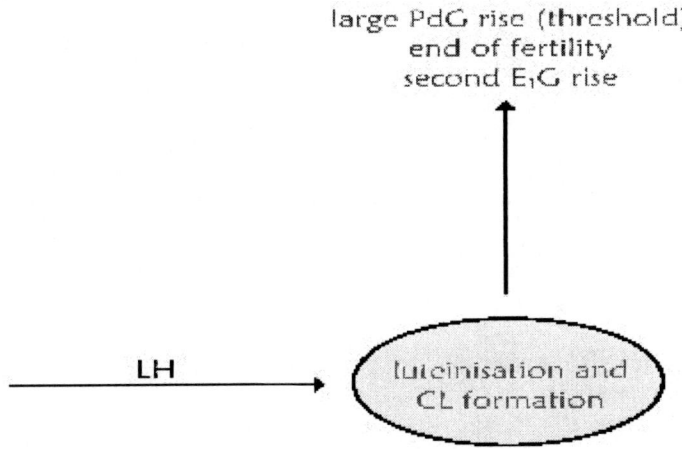

Figure 7. The fourth milestone - luteinization and corpus luteum formation.

> This first estrogen rise is therefore the chemical message which signals the beginning of fertility (Blackwell and Brown 1992)

3-6 days) after which a surge of luteinising hormone (LH) is released from the pituitary gland. This in turn triggers ovulation and converts the remnants of the follicle into a corpus luteum. As the LH surge begins there is a sharp drop in the excretion rate for estradiol (Hoff et al. 1983) and hence the characteristic mid-cycle estrogen peak day is observed. The day following the estrogen peak day is the most fertile day. If the LH surge is adequate and other factors are in place then the ovum is released and a small rise in progesterone (Hoff et al. 1983) or PdG is observed (Figure 6; the third milestone). This small PdG rise is a good indicator of ovulation and can be detected by the Ovarian Monitor.

> The E1G peak day and the first rise in PdG indicate the most fertile day of the cycle.

The fourth milestone follows if the LH surge is of sufficient magnitude and lasts long enough to cause luteinisation of the theca and granulosa cells which remain behind in the remnants of the follicle (Figure 7). These remnants become the corpus luteum and its estab-

Fifth Milestone

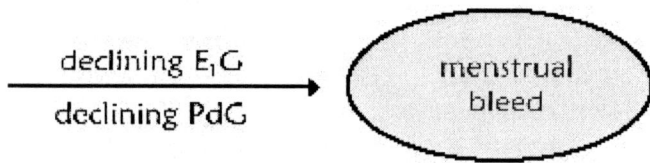

Normal luteal phase 11-16 days
PdG exceeds 10 µmol/24 hours

Figure 8 The fifth milestone - next menstrual bleed.

lishment as a functioning entity is essential to support any possible fertilized ova. Associated with corpus luteum establishment in the luteal phase is a huge increase in progesterone (Hoff et al. 1983) and a large associated increase in urinary PdG. Also associated with these events are the mucus peak symptom and the BBT rise.

A threshold level has been found using timed urine samples for this PdG rise which applies to all women and it is the preferred end-of fertility marker in our experience (Blackwell et al. 1998).

The final milestone (Figure 8) occurs if pregnancy does not take place. The estrogen and progesterone levels decline and the next menstrual bleed follows. If the interval between the day of the estrogen peak and the first day of bleeding is 11-16 days the cycle is classified as fertile and capable of sustaining a pregnancy should it have occurred—that is—a fertile ovulatory cycle. For a fully fertile ovulatory cycle these milestones must occur in the correct sequence at the correct times and be of appropriate magnitude and duration.

An example of a normal ovulatory cycle (which of course must show all of the milestones) obtained during the correlations of the Ovarian Monitor with reference radioimmunoassy results from the World Health Organisation reference laboratory at Hammersmith in London is shown in the next figure (Figure 9). This pattern has been well documented by many workers (for example see Collins, 1989). Day one is the first day of bleeding and the hormone values may still

Eavesdropping on the Ovary

be falling during the first day or two of the cycle. The low E1G values (below 100 nmol/24 hours) show that there is no major functioning follicle present and correspond to the basic infertile pattern of the Ovulation Method Billings (OM(B)) signifying the early safe days. The E1G values then begin to rise (on day 11 the first milestone occurs) which shows that a follicle (or group of follicles) has commenced its rapid growth phase and also corresponds to the onset of the mucus symptom (which signalled the beginning of fertility on cycle day 9). The E1G levels then continue to increase at a rate of about 140% per day to reach an E1G peak within 4-6 days (cycle day 15) and then they fall dramatically (milestone 2). This fall in E1G values shows that the rapid growth phase has ended but it occurs irrespective of whether the follicle is progressing to ovulation 24-36 hours later (a possibly

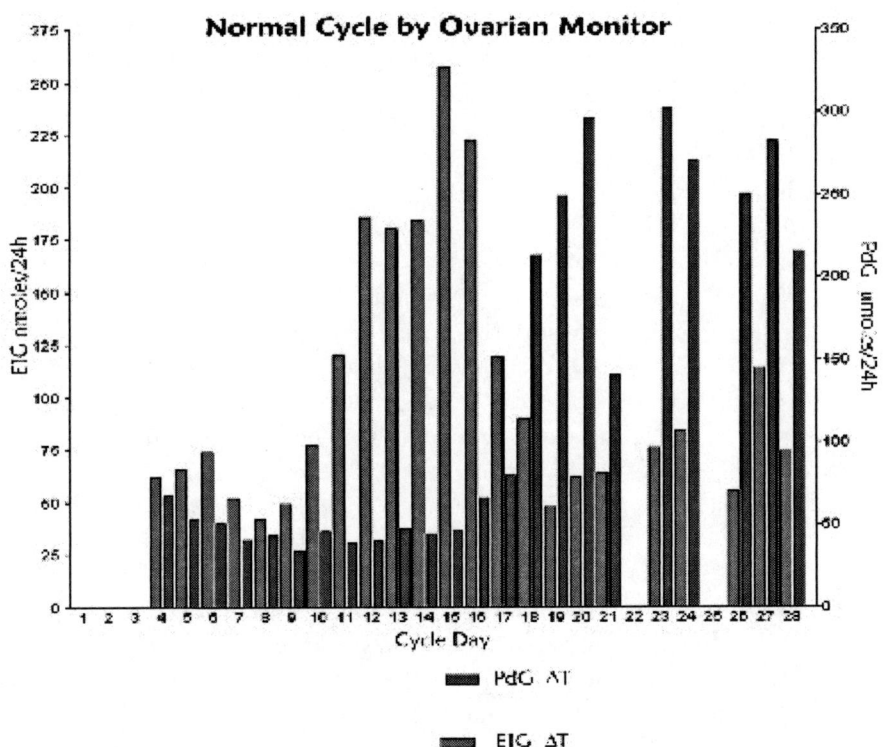

Figure 9. Typical ovulatory cycle monitored at home with the Ovarian Monitor. Cycle 022A2 from WHO study #90905.

fertile cycle) or to death by atresia (an infertile cycle). The E1G peak is therefore an ambiguous marker.

However, whether ovulation is occurring is shown clearly and unambiguously by the PdG values. We appear to be the only ones who utilizes this excellent marker (Blackwell et al. 1998) and believe that the failure of others to do so is a result of not using corrections for fluctuations in urine volume coupled with a lack of appreciation of the fact that the PdG rise is biphasic (Hoff et al. 1983). The PdG levels are uniformly low during the follicular phase but, if ovulation is occurring, they begin to rise at the time of the E1G peak (cycle day 16). Although the pre-ovulatory rise in PdG is small it is clearly identified by the Monitor in most cycles and is used routinely in Melbourne as a marker for ovulation. Ovulation occurs as the PdG values are passing through 4-5 μmol/24 hours and after ovulation the PdG values rise rapidly (milestone 4). This rise is quantitatively the largest hormonal change seen during the ovulatory cycle and levels reaching (or exceeding) 7 μmol/24 hours (the PdG cut-off) show that ovulation will not occur again in that cycle and that the post-ovulatory infertile days have commenced. The PdG threshold day was day 18 in this cycle. Hence, the fertile window extended from day 11 to day 17 or for 7 days with day 16 being the most fertile day. This shows one of the important reasons for correcting the urinary hormonal data for fluctuations in urine volume. There is a very small gap in time between the most fertile day and the end of the fertile window. Hence, the PdG assay used must be robust; accurate, reproducible and calibrated in absolute terms to read the true value in different cycles from different women. The luteal phase length was 13 days which when coupled with the fact that the PdG levels exceeded 10 μmol/24 hours demonstrates that this was a normal ovulatory cycle.

This information is most important for defining the post-ovulatory infertile days and allows intercourse to be resumed as soon as the PdG values reach, or exceed, 7 μmol/24 hours (Blackwell et al. 1998). The importance of providing accurate and robust PdG assays which allow these and other states to be recognised with certainty cannot be overemphasised. Most people equate the E1G rise and the mucus symptom with fertility; this is not strictly correct. They equate with fertility only when followed by ovulation as shown by the PdG rise, the peak mucus symptom or the BBT rise. It should be noted that the

PdG threshold and the BBT shift are the only positive indicators that ovulation has already occurred. All others, including the LH peak, the mucus peak and the E1G peak days are presumptive indicators only. When pregnancy occurs, the E1G and PdG values remain elevated and continue to rise. Thus, the E1G and PdG results provide all the information required on ovarian activity and also, by inference, on pituitary activity.

The above pattern (Figure 9) defines the essential features of the fertile ovulatory menstrual cycle. The E1G values may differ for different women but they are usually reproducible for the same woman. On the basis of these patterns rules can be defined, for the mucus symptoms and for the BBT for the achievement or avoidance of pregnancy. If all women at all times during their reproductive lives kept to this pattern of regular ovulatory activity, avoidance or achievement of pregnancy would be easy. However, the timing of the events will differ from cycle to cycle and from woman to woman. When considering NFP, most people think only in terms of the ovulatory cycle because this is the most common type of ovarian activity during the reproductive years. Unfortunately, other forms of ovarian activity can occur. No method of NFP is adequate unless allowance is made for this in the rules. These other forms of ovarian activity are completely normal responses to the environment to ensure that reproduction only occurs under favourable conditions. Professor Brown calls the total range of possible ovarian activities the Continuum.

The Ovarian Monitor

The Ovarian Monitor is a simple device that can be used for monitoring of the ovary at home. To do this it measures the levels of estrone glucuronide and pregnanediol glucuronide in timed urine specimens (Brown et al. 1989). The Monitor has been developed over the past sixteen years and at each stage it has been validated against reference assays or by similarly rigid criteria (Brown et al. 1988, 1989; Brown et al. 1968; Brown et al. 1978; Barrett and Brown 1970) and more recently by a World Health Organisation study (Blackwell et al. 2003). The Monitor consists of a simple colorimeter (Figure 10) and one assay tube which measures estrone glucuronide as a marker for the beginning of the potentially fertile phase plus a second assay tube which measures pregnanediol glucuronide as the end marker. The scientific basis of the Monitor has been published elsewhere (Brown et al., 1988, 1989) and will be reviewed in the accompanying paper. We can state that the home Ovarian Monitor gives values for PdG which are as accurate as the best available methods and that it gives values for E1G which are a little higher than our reference methods.

It is important to note that the physiological parameter which describes fertility is the excretion rate (amount per time) of the ovarian hormones. However, most measurements are in fact made as concentrations (amount per volume) and as a result the information from the ovary is degraded if the daily fluctuations in urine volume are not corrected. The variations in urine volume and concentration with time are so great that expressing the results in concentration units

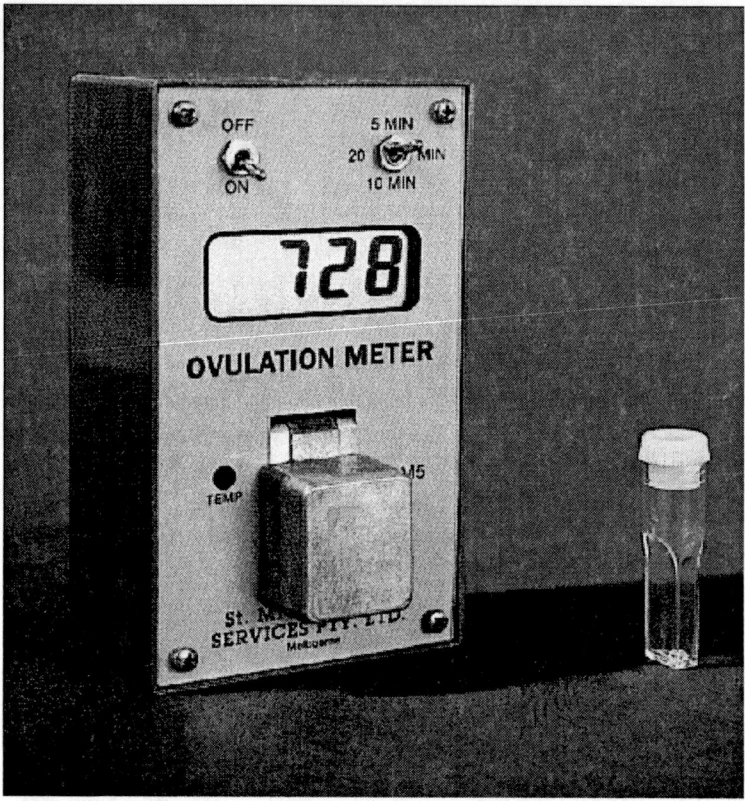

Figure 10. Picture of mark V Ovarian Monitor and an Ovarian Monitor assay tube showing its constituents.

without correcting for these variations gives meaningless information which may completely mask the daily changes in hormone levels being measured. This is particularly true for the PdG measurements where the cut-off value may be reached only a few hours after ovulation as discussed earlier. For example, Figure 11 shows a comparison of E1G and PdG data for the same cycle collected with and without correction

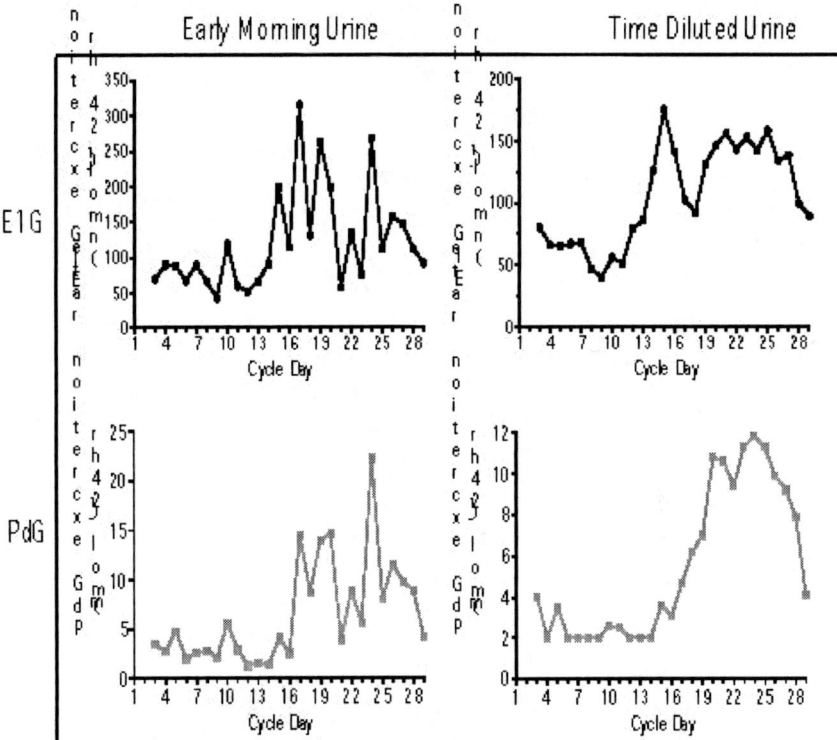

Figure 11. Comparison of E1G and PdG data for the same cycle collected with and without correction for urine volume.

for urine volume. For the E1G data taken from early morning urines (EMU) the pattern is not clear. Multiple peaks are seen and the E1G peak day is registered as day 17 instead of correctly as day 15 using timed urine data. For the PdG measurements the EMU data give an apparent PdG rise on day 17 (the same day as the E1G peak for the EMU data) whereas the true threshold day was day 19 (PdG > 7 μmol/24 hours). This is a serious discrepancy since day 17 is likely to be the most fertile day of this cycle and the EMU data would show the end of fertility (falsely) as day 17. It is not be clear from the EMU data what other signal could be used as the end of fertility. In marked contrast the timed urine data gives very clear patterns and the day of the beginning of fertility, the peak time of fertility and the day marking the beginning of the post-ovulatory infertile period are unambiguously defined. For this reason we have always used timed specimens of urine for our assays which now are either overnight or 3 hour collections. This reduces the time between the observation of ovarian activity and obtaining the hormone result. The data are still expressed as excretion per 24 hours. The full potential of hormonal monitoring can only be realised if correction for variation in urine volume is undertaken. Hence, the question must be asked whether the information obtained is worth the effort involved. We believe the answer is an emphatic yes.

The Continuum
(as described by Professor James B. Brown)

The major use of the Monitor has been as a research tool to sort out the Continuum, particularly the difficult cycles and to identify the infertile cycles as they are happening so that they can be used in their entirety. However, the insights given by the enormous body of information (mostly unpublished) now available have practical consequences for NFP which can help clients and teachers and persuade authorities of the rigorous scientific nature of modern NFP. The Continuum is presented as a sequence of the possible patterns of E1G and PdG values which have been found to occur. Professor Brown is currently publishing this concept.

Anovular cycles

1. The first stage of the continuum is a state of amenorrhea where there is no ovarian activity at all and the E1G and PdG values remain uniformly low. This is because there is no rise in FSH (no milestone one) and the situation may be permanent or temporary and may be followed by the development of a follicle which ovulates (shown by a rise and subsequent peak in the rate of E1G excretion and an

associated rise in PdG). This is one of the causes of a prolonged pre-ovulatory phase.

2. From a hormonal perspective, the next stage in the Continuum is the anovulatory cycle where E1G rises but PdG does not and there are two forms of this. The most common shows an E1G rise and fall indicating that a follicle has developed (milestone one achieved) as in the pre-ovulatory phase of the normal cycle, but the E1G rise has not triggered the LH surge (milestone 2 is not achieved). Hence the follicle does not ovulate but dies by atresia, giving rise to an E1G peak, but there is no rise in PdG values. Bleeding usually (but not always) follows the E1G fall – this is oestrogen withdrawal bleeding.

3. The second type of anovulatory cycle shows an estrogen rise which reaches a plateau, usually lower than the pre-ovulatory peak and the values remain at this plateau for a variable period of time. Bleeding usually occurs eventually as a breakthrough phenomenon but again there is no rise in PdG values. This type of anovulatory cycle is caused by a defect in the negative feedback mechanism (Brown 1978). This type of cycle can also be followed by a fertile ovulatory cycle with no interruption which often follows closely after the breakthrough bleed. This is the reason for the NFP rules which apply following mid-cycle bleeding.

Cycles with rising PdG values less than 6 μmol/24 hours

The next stages in the Continuum involve cycles for which there is a rise in the PdG values. The first of these types is the cycle with an unruptured luteinized follicle. In this case the E1G values rise and fall as in the anovulatory cycle and LH is released in insufficient amounts to initiate ovulation, but sufficient to cause some luteinization of the folllicle (we have almost got to milestone 3). Thus the PdG values rise after the E1G fall but do not reach the levels indicative of ovulation. It is important to understand that all of these stages where the PdG values do not exceed 6 μmol/24 hours can be followed by ovulation without an intervening bleed, or a bleed may lead directly into a fertile ovulatory response. NFP allows for this by stating that woman may be fertile during bleeding and distinguishes between the peak mucus symptom and a patch of mucus which only indicates the presence of a follicle.

Cycles with PdG values > 7µmol/24 hours

The next stage of the Continuum is ovulation (milestone 3 is achieved) but followed by a deficient or short luteal phase. In both these stages the PdG values rise above 7 µmol/24 hours but for the deficient luteal phase they do not rise above 9 µmol/24 hours. In the short luteal phase the PdG values do exceed 9 µmol/24 hours but the luteal phase only lasts 10 days, or less. Both these stages are infertile in that the luteal phase is insufficient to support a pregnancy but neither will be followed by a fertile ovulation without intervening bleeding. However, from the day on which the PdG values exceed 7 µmol/24 hours the cycle is infertile until the next bleed. That is, the luteal phase infertile period is indicated absolutely by the PdG threshold value. The dividing line between the unruptured luteinised follicle and the deficient luteal phase is not definite.

Ovulatory cycles

The final stage in the Continuum is the fully fertile ovulatory cycle but even this has degrees of hormone values and degrees of fertility. The minimum hormone requirements for a fully fertile ovulatory cycle are defined above, but at these minimum levels fertility is low with conception rates of 25% per cycle. Higher E1G and PdG values (PdG up to 36 µmol/24 hours) are more common and these are associated with higher conception rates of 70% per cycle. Still higher values 2 times the normal can be induced by the use of clomiphene and higher values again (3-5 times normal) by the use of gonadotrophins. Such enhanced levels produce a state of high fertility with the possibility of multiple pregnancy and provide a 47% conception rate per cycle in patients with longstanding unexplained infertility.

The stages of the Continuum are presented as an ordered sequence in which the PdG values increase from baseline to the high levels in stimulated cycles. This progression, from amenorrhea to ovulatory cycles, is seen during the year before and the three years after menarche (Brown et al. 1978) and during the return to fertility postpartum and during breast feeding (Brown et al. 1985). A regression back through the continuum is seen as women approach the menopause (Brown et al. 1981), in women with dysfunctional uterine bleeding, in women using oral contraception, in athletes and in any circumstance involving mental stress or loss of weight.

In general the changes through the Continuum are unpredictable, some stages may be skipped and a fully fertile ovulation can occur at any time. The stages of the Continuum need to be understood for optimum pregnancy avoidance and achievement. Confusion in symptoms caused by the Continuum is the main cause for risk taking in NFP and therefore unplanned pregnancies. The existence of the Continuum means that the interpretation of NFP observations will never be simple. In theory all possible positions on the continuum frame can be traversed by a cycle and these can be recognised easily by a simple measurement of E1G and PdG on a single urine sample. Daily testing will most likely be necessary to sort out the state of the continuum and currently this is only possible with the Ovarian Monitor or the ClearPlan Easy Fertility Monitor.

In summary, navigation through the continuum is achieved by three simple rules. A rise in E1G excretion rate above a woman's baseline level signifies the presence of a dominant follicle and hence potential fertility. A subsequent fall in E1G levels signifies possible ovulation or at least luteinization and must be tested for by the PdG excretion rate. If this equals or exceeds the threshold the post-ovulatory infertile time has arrived. Other stages in the continuum can be recognized by the absolute magnitude of the PdG levels. Application of the hormone values and use of the Monitor (Brown et al. 1991) will be described in the accompanying paper.

Acknowledgements

I wish to acknowledge the assistance over many years of my friends and colleagues Professor James Brown, Dr Meg Smith, Joanne Holmes, Gill Barker all of Melbourne and my students from Palmerston North, Yinqiu Wu, Mark Smales, Delwyn Cooke, Bryce Cummock, Zhao Zhang, Treena Blythe and Simone Flight.

Disclaimer

The material presented in this paper is based largely on information and data generously provided by Professor James Brown from Melbourne, Australia. In particular, the concept of the continuum is entirely from Professor Brown. Many of the figures are adapted from the Melbourne work with permission and from the WHO sponsored study of the Ovarian Monitor. The opinions expressed are the authors but result from many hours of discussion with Professor Brown. Any errors of interpretation are my responsibility.

Bibliography

Blackwell, L.F., and Brown, J.B. 1992. "Application of time-series analysis for the recognition of increases in urinary estrogens as markers for the beginning of the potentially fertile period." *Steroids* 57: 554-562.

Blackwell, L.F., Cooke, D.G., and Brown, J.B. 1998. "Definition of the potentially fertile period from urinary steroid excretion rates. Part II. A threshold value for pregnanediol glucuronide as a marker for the end of the potentially fertile period in the human menstrual cycle." *Steroids* 63: 5-13.

Blackwell, L.F., Brown, J.B., Vigil, P., Gross, B.A., Sufi, S., and d'Arcangues, C. 2003. "Hormonal monitoring of ovarian activity using the Ovarian Monitor, Part I. Validation of home and laboratory results obtained during ovulatory cycles by comparison with radioimmunoassay." *Steroids* 68: 465-476. Collins, W.P. 1989. "Biochemical indices of potential fertility." *International Journal of Gynecology and Obstetrics* Supplement 1: 35-43.

Brown, J.B., MacLeod, S.C., Macnaughtan, C., Smith, M.A., and Smyth, B. 1968. "A rapid method for measuring oestrogens in urine using a semi-automatic extractor." *Journal of Endocrinology* 42: 5-15.

Barrett, S.A. and Brown, J.B. 1970. "An evaluation of the method of Cox for the rapid analysis of pregnanediol in urine by gas liquid chromatography." *Journal of Endocrinology* 47: 471-480.

Brown, J.B. 1978. "Pituitary control of ovarian function – concepts derived from gonadotrophin therapy." *Australian & New Zealand Journal of Obstetrics & Gynaecology* 18: 46-54.

Brown, J.B., Harrisson, P. and Smith, M.A. 1978. "Oestrogen and pregnanediol excretion throughout childhood, menarche and first ovulation." *Journal of Biosocial Science* Supplement 5: 43-62.

Brown, J.B., Beischer, N.A. and Quin, M.A. 1981. "Urinary oestrogens and pregnancy." *Journal of Endocrinology* Supplement 89: 95P-102P.

Brown, J.B., Harrisson, P. and Smith, M.A. 1985. "A study of returning fertility after childbirth and during lactation by measurement of urinary oestrogen and pregnanediol excretion and cervical mucus production." *Journal of Biosocial Science* – Supplement 9: 5-23.

Brown, J.B., Blackwell, L.F., Cox, R.I., Holmes, J.M., and Smith, M.A. 1988. "Chemical and homogeneous enzyme immunoassay methods for the measurment of oestrogens and pregnanediol and their glucuronides in urine." *Progress in Biological and Clinical Research* 285: 119-138.

Brown, J.B., Blackwell, L.F., Homes, J.M., and Smyth, K. 1989. "New assays for identifying the fertile period." *International Journal of Gynecology and Obstetrics* Supplement 1: 111-122.

Brown, J.B., Holmes, J.M., and Barker. G. 1991. "Use of the home ovarian monitor in pregnancy avoidance." *American Journal of Obstetrics and Gynecology* Supplement 185: 2008-2011.

Doody, M.C., Gibbons, W.E. and Zamah, N.M. 1987. "Linear regression analysis of ultrasound folliclular growth series: satistical relationship of growth rate and calculated data of growth onset to total grwoth period." *Fertility and Sterility* 47: 436-439.

Hoff, J.D., Quigley, M.E., and Yen, S.C.C. 1983. "Hormonal dynamics at mid-cycle: A reevaluation." *Journal of Clinical Endocrinology and Metabolism* 57: 792-796.

Gore, M.A., Nayudu, P.L., and Vlaisavljevic, V. 1997. "Attaining dominance in vivo: distinguishing dominant from challenger follicles in humans." *Human Reproduction* 12: 2741-2747.

McNatty, K.P. 1981. "Hormonal correlates of follicular development in the human ovary." *Australian Journal of Biological Science* 34: 249-268.

Thornton, S.J., Pepperell, R.J., and Brown, J.B. 1990. "Home monitoring of gonadotrophin ovulation induction using the Ovarian Monitor." *Fertility and Sterility* 54: 1076-1081.

SPECIAL CONTRIBUTION

Executive summary: Stages of Reproductive Aging Workshop (STRAW)

Michael R. Soules, M.D.,[a] Sherry Sherman, Ph.D.,[b] Estella Parrott, M.D., M.P.H.,[c] Robert Rebar, M.D.,[a] Nanette Santoro, M.D.,[d] Wulf Utian, M.D., Ph.D.,[e] and Nancy Woods, R.N., Ph.D.[e]

American Society for Reproductive Medicine, National Institute on Aging, National Institute of Child Health and Human Development, Albert Einstein College of Medicine, and the North American Menopause Society

Received and accepted August 24, 2001.
Correspondence: Michael R. Soules, M.D., 4225 Roosevelt Way NE, #305, Seattle, Washington 98105 (FAX: 206-685-7818; E-mail: msoules@u.washington.edu).
[a] Division of Reproductive Endocrinology and Infertility, American Society for Reproductive Medicine.
[b] Clinical Endocrinology and Osteoporosis Research, National Institute on Aging, National Institutes of Health.
[c] Reproductive Medicine Gynecology Program, National Institute of Child Health and Human Development, National Institutes of Health.
[d] Division of Reproductive Endocrinology and Infertility, Albert Einstein College of Medicine.
[e] North American Menopause Society.

0015-0282/-1900/$20.00
PII S0015-0282(01)02909-0

The Stages of Reproductive Aging Workshop (STRAW) was held in Park City, Utah, on July 23 and 24, 2001. There were 27 invited participants, most of whom had extensive clinical or research experience in reproductive aging in women. The sponsors were the American Society for Reproductive Medicine (ASRM), the National Institute on Aging (NIA), the National Institute of Child Health and Human Development (NICHD), and the North American Menopause Society (NAMS). The purpose of the workshop was to address the absence of a relevant staging system for female reproductive aging and to discuss the confusing current nomenclature for the premenopause.

The workshop consisted of focused presentations on menstrual cyclicity, endocrinology, pelvic anatomy, symptoms in other organ systems, nomenclature, fertility, and clinical and basic research gaps in relation to reproductive aging. A panel discussion and a group discussion followed each presentation. Later, breakout groups sought agreement on the practical utility of different signs and symptoms for a staging system. Subsequently, the leaders of each breakout groups presented their recommendations to all participants, and these recommendations were melded into a combined staging system (Fig. 1). Each point in the proposed staging system was accepted by at least a supermajority (70%) of the participants (there was unanimity on most points).

Women neither initiate reproductive function (puberty) nor end it (menopause) at a particular chronological age. Both puberty and the menopausal transition are dynamic periods for the reproductive axis, during which development or senescence occurs relatively quickly. While there is a useful staging system for puberty (the Tanner/Marshall system [(1)]), a similar staging system for late reproductive function has not been developed. The need for a staging system has been most apparent to the biomedical research community, but the intended audience of the workshop also included two secondary groups: health practitioners and the public. The specific goals of the reproductive aging workshop were to [1] develop a relevant and useful staging system, [2] revise the nomenclature, and [3] identify knowledge gaps (both clinical and basic) that should be addressed by the research community.

BACKGROUND AND SIGNIFICANCE

Aging can be defined as the natural progression of changes in structure and function that occur with the passage of time in the absence of known disease. The female reproductive axis essentially comprises the hypothalamic–pituitary–ovarian axis and the müllerian-derived structures (e.g., the uterus). The reproductive axis ages to a nonfunctional state (menopause) much earlier than do the other organ systems, at a time when a woman is otherwise healthy. The basis of reproductive senescence in women is oocyte depletion in the ovary. A woman is endowed at birth with a finite number of oocytes that are arrested in prophase I of meiosis. Reproductive aging consists of a steady loss of oocytes through atresia or ovulation, which does not necessarily occur

874

FIGURE 1

The STRAW staging system.

Stages:	-5	-4	-3	-2	-1	0	+1	+2
Terminology:	Reproductive			Menopausal Transition		Final Menstrual Period (FMP)	Postmenopause	
	Early	Peak	Late	Early	Late*		Early*	Late
				Perimenopause				
Duration of Stage:	variable			variable		(a) 1 yr	(b) 4 yrs	until demise
Menstrual Cycles:	variable to regular	regular		variable cycle length (>7 days different from normal)	≥2 skipped cycles and an interval of amenorrhea (≥60 days)		none	
Endocrine:	normal FSH		↑ FSH	↑ FSH			↑ FSH	

*Stages most likely to be characterized by vasomotor symptoms   ↑ = elevated

Soules. Executive Summary of STRAW. Fertil Steril 2001.

at a constant rate. The relatively wide age range (42–58 years) for menopause in normal women seems to indicate that women are either endowed with a highly variable number of oocytes or the rate of oocyte loss varies greatly.

Reproductive aging is a natural process that begins at birth and proceeds as a continuum. Clearly it is a *process* and not an *event*, and the end (menopause) is much easier to define than the beginning. Knowing that chronological age is a very poor indicator of reproductive aging, the purpose of a staging system would be to identify what point a given woman has reached in the process of reproductive aging.

SUBJECTS

Until recently, interest in and studies of reproductive aging have been lacking. An understanding of the pattern of reproductive senescence in normal healthy women is just now emerging. Most of the current medical information in this field has come from studies of a narrow segment of the population (white women of mid- to upper socioeconomic means). However, the signs and symptoms of reproductive aging appear to differ by race, ethnicity, culture, geographic region, and socioeconomic status. Given these considerations, the workshop concentrated on developing a staging system for all healthy women who age spontaneously to a natural menopause.

Although all women will probably experience similar signs and symptoms as they develop ovarian failure, we recommend not applying this staging system in women who smoke cigarettes, those at the extremes of body weight (body mass index <18 kg/m^2 or >30 kg/m^2), those who do heavy aerobic exercise (>10 h/wk), those who have had a hysterectomy, or those who have abnormal uterine (e.g., fibroids) or ovarian anatomy (e.g., endometrioma).

CRITERIA FOR AN IDEAL STAGING SYSTEM

An ideal staging system would have the following characteristics:

- It would rely only on objective data, because symptoms are inherently subjective.
- It would use only reliable tests that are relatively inexpensive and readily available.
- It would allow women to be placed in the appropriate stage prospectively.
- Inclusion in one stage would preclude placement in another stage.

THE STAGING SYSTEM

A dominant pattern for reproductive senescence has been identified that forms the basis for the recommended staging system (Fig. 1). However, not all healthy women will follow this pattern. While most normal women will progress from one stage to the next, some will "see-saw" between stages or skip a stage altogether.

The workshop participants considered several potential components of a staging system: menstrual cycles, endocrine and biochemical factors, fertility, signs and symptoms in other organ systems, and uterine/ovarian anatomy. Each component was discussed separately. The anchor for the staging system is the final menstrual period (FMP). Five stages occur before the FMP (Fig. 1); the age range and duration for each of these stages varies. The staging system that was developed at the workshop has seven stages; five precede and two follow the final menstrual period. Stages −5 to −3 encompass the reproductive interval; stages −2 and −1 are the menopausal transition; and stages 1 and 2 are the postmenopause (Fig. 1).

Menstrual Cyclicity

After menarche (entry into stage −5) it usually takes several years for regular menstrual cycles to become established. Menstrual periods should then occur every 21 to 35 days for a number of years (stages −4 and −3). There is no clear demarcation between stages −5 to −3, since fertility increases and decreases gradually and imperceptibly over many years. A woman's menstrual cycles remain regular in stage −2 (early menopausal transition), but the duration changes by 7 days or more (e.g., her regular cycles are now every 24 instead of 31 days). Stage −1 (late menopausal transition) is characterized by two or more skipped menstrual cycles and at least one intermenstrual interval of 60 days or more. Although the workshop participants recognized that duration and amount of menstrual flow often change during the menopausal transition, these changes were considered to be highly variable and were therefore not included in the staging system. Several prospective longitudinal studies of menstrual cyclicity have documented that many women are poor historians of even their recent menstrual history; it is recommended that investigators and clinicians confirm menstrual histories by asking women to keep prospective menstrual calendars. Sonography or other imaging of the uterus should be done at baseline and periodically (every 2 to 3 years) to document that uterine bleeding is due to hormonal changes and not uterine pathology (e.g., leiomyoma or adenomyosis).

Endocrinology

Only rudimentary knowledge of the endocrinology of the menstrual cycle is needed to use the staging system. An elevated FSH level is the first measurable sign of reproductive aging. This initial elevation in FSH level is most prominent in the early follicular phase of the cycle; a single venous blood sample should be obtained between cycle days 2 and 5 (the first day of flow is day 1) and subsequently assayed for FSH and estradiol. Serum FSH immunoassays are readily available and relatively inexpensive. The initial elevation in the late reproductive stage −3 is subtle; while clinicians often use 10 mIU/mL as the cutoff value, in the research setting it would be best to determine the actual level for a particular laboratory in a young control sample from stage −4 (peak reproductive time). An elevated FSH level would be an early follicular phase level that exceeds 2 SDs of the mean level for a sample of normal women of peak reproductive age (25–30 years). In the late reproductive stage, the estradiol level in the early follicular phase is either normal or elevated; if it is elevated, it can suppress what otherwise would be an elevated FSH level and, therefore, the FSH level should only be interpreted in the context of a simultaneously measured estradiol level. (An estradiol level >80 pg/ml is often considered to be elevated.) An elevated FSH level in a single cycle is significant and is sufficient to categorize a woman as stage −3; an elevated level does not need to be repeated. However, a normal FSH level in a 40- to 45-year-old woman with regular cycles will be elevated in a preceding or subsequent cycle about 30% of the time. Therefore, in this group, it is recommended that FSH be measured a second time if the first value is normal. It is recognized that FSH levels gradually increase throughout the menopausal transition, but levels vary greatly and it would be difficult to identify meaningful cut-off levels for stages −3 to +1.

Other reproductive hormones undergo significant and predictable changes during the menopausal transition. Estradiol levels eventually decrease, LH levels change later than FSH levels but gradually increase, and progesterone levels decrease as ovulation ceases. However, the variability of each of these hormone changes is high, thus diminishing their utility for a staging system. A fall in inhibin B is the basis for the FSH rise with ovarian aging, but use of this difficult and relatively unavailable assay would not contribute to this staging system. Serum hormone assays are more readily available and validated, but urinary hormone assays provide a more integrated picture of hormone secretion over time. In the research setting, it may be useful to use serum assays when cycles are regular and urine assays in the late menopausal transition (stage −1) when cycles are irregular. Normative data are not as readily available for urinary assays as for serum assays.

Symptoms

Some women start to experience various symptoms during the late reproductive phase (stage −3), including vasomotor symptoms, breast tenderness, insomnia, migraines, and premenstrual dysphoria. In addition, genital atrophic symptoms and problems in sexual function can occur in the late menopausal transition and beyond. Not all women have symptoms as they transition to the menopause, and women with symptoms experience them in different combinations and at different intensities. Quantification of these symptoms is difficult because they are subjective by nature. It has been observed that symptomology varies markedly among ethnic groups, cultures, socioeconomic groups, and climates. Furthermore, the symptoms do not track closely with the menstrual cycle or endocrine changes during the menopausal transition. Vasomotor symptoms are the most frequent and prominent of the menopausal symptoms; women in stages −1 and +1 frequently experience onset or increased intensity of such symptoms.

Fertility

A woman's peak fertility occurs in her mid- to late twenties, after which it progressively decreases until menopause (stage −4 to −1). The loss of fertility is the first sign of reproductive aging that precedes the monotropic increase in FSH level and changes in menstrual cyclicity. However, fertility was not included in the staging system because relative fertility in an individual is nearly impossible to measure and is codependent on the fertility of the male partner.

Imaging

The workshop considered imaging of the pelvic organs by various methods (e.g., ultrasonography, magnetic resonance imaging, and computed tomography) for their potential to contribute to a staging system. For practical purposes, the best imaging method is sonography. Uterine sonography did not seem applicable to the staging system, but it may be used to rule out uterine pathology as a cause of uterine bleeding. Ultrasonography can also rule out ovarian pathology (e.g., dermoid), which may affect reproductive aging.

Ovarian sonography, specifically antral follicle (2–10 mm) counts, appears to be promising for use in a future revision of the staging system. The number of antral follicles in the ovary does not vary over the menstrual cycle, correlates well with chronological age, and probably reflects the size of the reserve pool of primordial follicles. However, studies of antral follicle counts in women during the menopausal transition are lacking.

NOMENCLATURE

The workshop participants recognized the current confusion and duplication in the nomenclature as applied to female reproductive senescence. The World Health Organization (WHO) has attempted to address these concerns on several occasions (most recently in 1996 [(2)]). The Council of Affiliated Menopause Societies (CAMS) convened a working group to further define the terminology in 1999 (3). The WHO and CAMS definitions generally have vague starting points and use terms that overlap, such as *premenopause, perimenopause, menopausal transition,* and *climacteric.* Our recommendations for a revision in the nomenclature are as follows.

Menopause: The anchor point that is defined after 12 months of amenorrhea following the FMP, which reflects a near complete but natural decrease in ovarian hormone secretion.

Menopausal transition: Stage −2 (early) and −1 (late) encompass the menopausal transition and are defined by menstrual cycle and endocrine changes. The menopausal transition begins with variation in menstrual cycle length in a woman who has a monotropic FSH rise and ends with the FMP (not able to be recognized until after 12 months of amenorrhea).

Postmenopause: Stage +1 (early) and +2 (late) encompass the postmenopause. The early postmenopause is defined as 5 years since the FMP. The participants agreed this interval is relevant because it encompasses a further dampening of ovarian hormone function to a permanent level as well as accelerated bone loss. Stage +1 was further subdivided into segment "a", the first 12 months after the FMP, and segment "b", the next 4 years. Stage +2 has a definite beginning but its duration varies, since it ends with death. Further divisions may be warranted as women live longer and more information is accumulated.

Perimenopause: Literally means "about or around the menopause." It begins with stage −2 and ends 12 months after the FMP. "The climacteric" is a popular but vague term that we recommend be used synonymously with perimenopause. Generally speaking, the terms *perimenopause* and *climacteric* should be used only with patients and in the lay press and not in scientific papers.

The success of the workshop will depend on whether investigators, clinicians, and others find this staging system and nomenclature useful. We believe that it is a distinct improvement over the current situation: a nonexistent staging system and confusing nomenclature. However, the participants recognize that this is a work in progress and expect to make revisions as more knowledge becomes available.

APPENDIX

STRAW Planning Committee

Michael R. Soules, M.D., Co-Chair: Professor and Director, Division of Reproductive Endocrinology and Infertility, Department of Obstetrics and Gynecology, University of Washington; President, American Society for Reproductive Medicine.

Sherry Sherman, Ph.D., Co-Chair: Director, Clinical Endocrinology and Osteoporosis Research, National Institute on Aging, National Institutes of Health.

Estella Parrott, M.D., M.P.H.: Program Director, Reproductive Medicine Gynecology Program, Center for Population Research, National Institute of Child Health and Human Development, National Institutes of Health.

Robert Rebar, M.D.: Associate Executive Director, American Society for Reproductive Medicine.

Nanette Santoro, M.D., Professor and Director, Division of Reproductive Endocrinology and Infertility, Albert Einstein College of Medicine.

Wulf Utian, M.D., Ph.D.: Professor Emeritus, Case Western Reserve University; Executive Director, North American Menopause Society.

Nancy Woods, R.N., Ph.D.: Dean, School of Nursing, Professor, Family and Child Nursing, University of Washington; Past President, North American Menopause Society.

STRAW PARTICIPANTS

Nancy Avis, Ph.D., Wake Forest University School of Medicine

Henry Burger, M.D., Monash University (Australia)

Sybil Crawford, Ph.D., University of Massachusetts

Lorraine Dennerstein, M.B.B.S., Ph.D., University of Melbourne (Australia)

Gregory F. Erickson, Ph.D., University of California, San Diego

Roger Gosden, Ph.D., McGill University (Canada)

Gail Greendale, M.D., University of California, Los Angeles

Sioban Harlow, Ph.D., University of Michigan

Kay Johannes, Ph.D., New England Research Institutes

Nancy Klein, M.D., University of Washington

Bill Lasley, Ph.D., University of California, Davis

James Liu, M.D., University of Cincinnati

Ellen Mitchell, R.N., Ph.D., University of Washington

Kathleen O'Connor, Ph.D., University of Washington

Mary Lake Polan, M.D., Ph.D., Stanford University

Jerilynn Prior, M.D., University of British Columbia (Canada)

John Randolph, Jr., M.D., University of Michigan

Nancy Reame, R.N., Ph.D., University of Michigan

Richard T. Scott, M.D., Reproductive Medicine Associates of New Jersey

Gerson Weiss, M.D., New Jersey Medical School

References

1. Marshall WA, Tanner JM. Variations in pattern of pubertal changes in girls. Arch Dis Childhood 1969;44:291.
2. WHO Scientific Group. Research on Menopause in the 1990s. Report of a WHO Scientific Group. WHO Technical Report Series 866. Geneva: WHO, 1996.
3. Utian WH. The International Menopause Society, Menopause-related terminology definitions. Climacteric 1999;2:284–6.

Contraception

Contraception 65 (2002) 333-338

Original research article

Efficacy of a new method of family planning: the Standard Days Method☆

Marcos Arévalo, Victoria Jennings*, Irit Sinai

Georgetown University, 3 PHC, 3800 Reservoir Rd., NW, Washington, DC 20007, USA

Received 19 November 2001; received in revised form 12 December 2001; accepted 12 December 2001

Abstract

The Standard Days Method is a fertility awareness-based method of family planning in which users avoid unprotected intercourse during cycle Days 8 through 19. A prospective multi-center efficacy trial was conducted to test, in a heterogeneous population, the contraceptive efficacy of the Standard Days Method. A total of 478 women, age 18–39 years, in Bolivia, Peru, and the Philippines, with self-reported cycles of 26–32 days, desiring to delay pregnancy at least one year were admitted to the study. A single decrement multi-censoring life table analysis of the data indicate a cumulative probability of pregnancy of 4.75% over 13 cycles of correct use of the method, and a 11.96% probability of pregnancy under typical use. This article describes the study and the results. Results suggest that despite its requirement that couples modify their sexual behavior when the woman is fertile, the Standard Days Method provides significant protection from unplanned pregnancy and is acceptable to couples in a wide range of settings. © 2002 Elsevier Science Inc. All rights reserved.

Keywords: Standard Days Method; Contraceptive efficacy; Fertility awareness

1. Introduction

A couple wanting to avoid or achieve pregnancy by timing intercourse needs to know when during her menstrual cycle the woman is most likely to become pregnant. They can do so by using a fertility awareness-based family planning method. The fertile window of the woman's menstrual cycle consists of approximately 6 days—the 5 days before ovulation and the day of ovulation, with variable probabilities of pregnancy for each day [1,2]. However, the timing of ovulation is variable both among women and across cycles of the same woman, with some women experiencing much greater variability than others [3]. A fertility awareness-based method that takes into account this variability could be a viable option for many couples. The Institute for Reproductive Health, Georgetown University,

---

☆ Support for conceptualizing the SDM, implementing the effectiveness study, and preparing this article was provided by the Institute for Reproductive Health, Department of Obstetrics and Gynecology at Georgetown University, Washington, DC, which is funded under a cooperative agreement HRN-A-00-97-11100-00 with the United States Agency for International Development (USAID).

* Corresponding author. Tel.: +1-202-687-1392; fax: +1-202-687-6846.

E-mail address: jenningv@georgetown.edu (V. Jennings).

proposed a fixed formula in which women who typically have menstrual cycles of 26 to 32 days consider themselves fertile during Days 8 through 19 (12 days) of their cycles. To prevent unplanned pregnancy, they avoid unprotected intercourse on those days [4].

Ideally, a woman using a fertility awareness-based method should be able to identify the 6 days of her fertile window, with neither "false positives" (i.e., days identified as fertile that actually are infertile), nor "false negatives" (i.e., days identified as infertile that actually are fertile) [5]. The technology necessary for this degree of accuracy, however, is not widely available or affordable, especially in developing countries. Balancing the need to provide effective protection from unplanned pregnancy while restricting the identified fertile period to as few days as possible, we developed the Standard Days Method (SDM), in which a woman considers herself potentially fertile on Days 8 through 19 of her menstrual cycle. If she does not want to become pregnant, she avoids unprotected intercourse on those days.

To develop the SDM, we applied various formulae (i.e., various numbers of days and various sets of days) to over 7500 menstrual cycles in an existing data set from the World Health Organization (WHO) [6]. The goal was to determine which formula provided the best balance between

0010-7824/02/$ – see front matter © 2002 Elsevier Science Inc. All rights reserved.
PII: S0010-7824(02)00288-3

length of the identified fertile period and efficacy in avoiding unplanned pregnancy. To accomplish this, we developed a computer simulation that took into account the variable probability of pregnancy on different cycle days before and including the probable day of ovulation as well as the variable probability of ovulation occurring on different cycle days.[1] The 8 through 19 formula provided maximum protection while minimizing the number of days of avoiding unprotected intercourse. We estimated that if women with cycles ranging 26 to 32 days had used the 8 through 19 formula and avoided unprotected intercourse on those days, the highest probability of pregnancy on any given day was only 0.007.

We then estimated that the method would be almost as effective for women who typically have cycles within the 26 through 32 day range but occasionally (no more than twice in a 12-month period) have a shorter or longer cycle. However, the 8 through 19 formula would be less effective for women who consistently have cycles shorter than 26 days or longer than 32 days. Nonetheless, even when all women and all cycles regardless of length were included in the computer simulation, the highest probability of pregnancy/intercourse on any given day was still only 0.011.

In designing this efficacy study, we followed the guidelines recommended by Trussell and Kost [7]. Data collection instruments, participant enrollment, and pregnancy definition were all influenced by those recommendations. Their guidelines also affected the way we analyzed the data and, thus the results presented in this article.

2. Materials and methods

A prospective, non-randomized, multi-center study to test the efficacy of the SDM was conducted among culturally diverse populations. Participants were enrolled from five sites in Bolivia (Trinidad), Peru (Juliaca and Lima), and the Philippines (La Trinidad and Tuba).

2.1. Study participants

A total of 478 women (married or living with a stable partner) were admitted to the study. All participants were between 18 and 39 years old (to minimize cycle variability and subfertility), had regular menstrual cycles (defined as recent history of most cycles between 26 and 32 days long, as determined by a screening protocol), were willing to avoid intercourse 12 consecutive days every cycle, and had partners willing to collaborate. Potential participants were screened for subfecundity, risk of sexually transmitted diseases, and contraindications of pregnancy.

2.2. Procedures

In all sites, the Institute for Reproductive Health trained 5 to 10 health workers (service providers) in the SDM and in study procedures. Method provision involved a counseling session in which the woman (or the couple, if her partner was available) was instructed in the SDM, and counseled on the importance of following the method recommendations to avoid pregnancy. She was invited to contact the provider with questions and to include her partner in any subsequent contact, as appropriate. To assist women in monitoring their cycles, the provider gave them a mnemonic device, a string of 32 beads in which each bead represents a day of the menstrual cycle. The first bead is red, representing the first day of menses; the next 6 beads are brown, representing the additional non-fertile days preceding the fertile window; the next 12 beads are white, representing days that should be considered fertile (8–19); and the remaining 13 beads are brown, again representing non-fertile days. The bead assembly also has a moveable, tight-fitting rubber ring that is used to mark the current day of the cycle. Women were instructed to place the ring on the red bead on the day their menses began and to move the ring one bead per day until their menses returned. They also were told that to avoid pregnancy, they should not have unprotected intercourse on the days the ring was on a white bead. If they had menstrual bleeding before Day 27 of the cycle (i.e., a cycle shorter than 26 days), or if their menses had not occurred by the day after they completed all 32 beads (i.e., a cycle longer than 32 days), they were instructed to contact their provider for further assessment and advice. Women who had two cycles outside the 26 through 32 day range during the study period were advised to use another method and were withdrawn from the study.[2] The mnemonic device, called CycleBeads, and its instructions are shown in Fig. 1.

Providers also were trained to collect the data needed for the study. The protocol, data collection instruments and consent form were approved by the Georgetown University Medical Center Institutional Review Board. Written, informed consent was obtained from all study participants.

In addition to using the CycleBeads to monitor their cycle days, for study purposes participants also marked the first day of their menses on a calendar and kept a coital log in which they also indicated the days they used another method (i.e., condom or withdrawal). Women in the study were interviewed each cycle, until they either completed 13 cycles or left the study for other reasons. During each interview, the interviewer reviewed the woman's completed coital log, checked the cycle day indicated on the calendar with the position of the ring on the CycleBeads, determined whether she continued to use the method (including reason for discontinuation, if applicable), and screened for possible pregnancy. Women who had not had their menses by Day 42 of their cycle were tested for pregnancy. If results were negative, they were followed until they tested positive or their menses returned. They were then exited from the study because of extremely irregular cycle length. Loss to follow-up was minimized by interviewing study participants in their homes and actively seeking out each participant, with a minimum of three attempts per cycle.

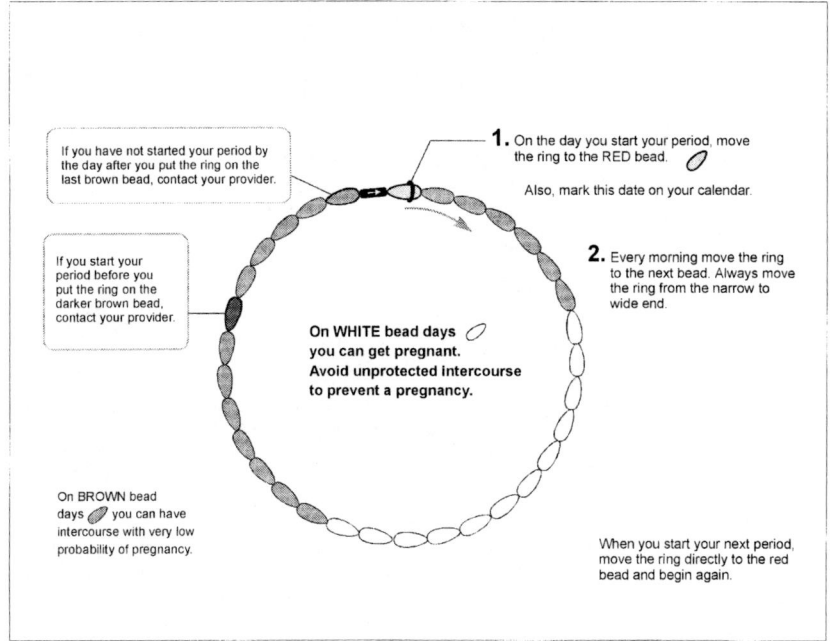

Fig. 1. CycleBeads and instructions for use.

2.3. Analysis

We used single-decrement multi-censoring life tables. Multi-censoring life tables allowed us to exclude some cycles from the analysis without censoring the woman contributing the cycles from the rest of the study [8]. We excluded cycles during which the participant did not have intercourse (0.35%) because there was no exposure to the risk of pregnancy. We also excluded cycles during which another method of family planning was used on days other than 8 through 19, which are identified as non-fertile by the SDM. These cycles were excluded because it is not possible to determine whether the woman was protected from pregnancy by the SDM only or by the other method.

3. Results

A total of 478 women were admitted into the trial, with a mean age of 29.4 years. Women in the study were drawn from urban, mixed urban/rural and rural sites. Lima was the largest city; study participants from La Trinidad (the Philippines), Trinidad (Bolivia), and Juliaca (Peru) lived in a variety of mixed urban/rural settings in these smaller cities; Tuba (the Philippines) was a rural site.

Participants' educational levels were relatively high: more than 90% of women had completed primary education. When asked to read simple instructions related to the method, only 9% of women either could not read them or had difficulty completing the task.

Almost all (98.9%) study participants had children, with a mean of 2.5 children per woman. Most participants had at least one child 2 years old or younger. As would be expected given the communities where they lived, almost 80% of study participants stated they were Catholic, although only one woman mentioned her religious beliefs as a factor in her choice of method.

There was significant variability among the sites with regard to previous use of family planning. Women living in more urban areas had more experience with hormonal contraceptives and intrauterine devices, while traditional methods were more common in rural areas. Although one-third of women were breastfeeding at admission, they met all study criteria, including having experienced at least three

Table 1
Profile of participants in the Standard Days Method efficacy study (n = 478)

Characteristic	Percent of participants
Study site	
Trinidad, Bolivia	11.5
Juliaca, Peru	21.3
Lima, Peru	21.1
La Trinidad, Philippines	21.3
Tuba, Philippines	24.7
Age at admission	
18–24	23.5
25–29	25.6
30–34	29.4
35–39	21.4
Parity	
No children	1.1
1–2 children	58.3
3–4 children	32.1
5 children or more	8.5
Education	
Completed primary education or lower	14.9
Some secondary education or higher	85.1
Occupation	
No income earning occupation	51.9
Agriculture	5.5
Sales	18.3
Blue collar job	15.3
White collar job	8.9
Ever use of family planning methods[a]	
None	9.6
Calendar	55.9
Withdrawal	37.0
Lactational Amenorreah (LAM)	1.3
Other natural methods	2.7
Barrier method	30.8
Intra Uterine Device	12.8
Hormonal method	30.0

[a] Figures add to more than 100% because many respondents specified more than one method.

Table 2
Reason for exiting from Standard Days Method efficacy study (n = 478)

Reason for exit	Percent of participants
Completed 13 cycles	45.6
Had 2 cycles out of the 26–32-day range[a]	28.0
Was told that a pregnancy would be high risk	0.2
Client did not like the method	0.2
Client did not trust the method	1.7
Partner did not like the method	2.1
Wanted to get pregnant	2.1
Exited for another voluntary reason	4.0
Lost to follow-up	7.1
Pregnant	9.0

[a] Includes also 25 clients who exited after just one cycle out of range. Of these, 12 clients had a cycle 42 days or longer, and 13 clients exited early because of an error.

regular cycles since the last birth. Almost half of study participants received an income from work outside the home. The client profile is shown in Table 1.

Of all women who entered the study, 46% completed 13 cycles of method use. Of those who did not complete 13 cycles, the largest group (28% of the total sample) corresponds to those who, following the study protocol, were removed from the study after they had two cycles outside the 26 through 32 day range (including 13 women erroneously exited after a single such cycle) or experienced a single cycle longer than 42 days. Throughout 13 cycles of method use, very few women (4%) left the study because they or their partner did not like or trust the method. Reasons for leaving the study are presented in Table 2.

A total of 4035 cycles were contributed by the 478 study participants. Correct method use (no intercourse on Days 8–19) was reported in 92% of cycles. In an additional 5% of cycles, intercourse did occur, but with use of another method (condom or withdrawal). Unprotected intercourse occurred in only 3% of cycles. A total of only 43 pregnancies occurred during the study. Predictably, most (65%) of the pregnancies occurred during cycles in which the woman reported unprotected intercourse during Days 8 through 19 (days identified as fertile by the method). Only 15 study participants became pregnant in cycles in which no intercourse was reported during Days 8–19. Most pregnancies occurred during the first cycles of method use (42% of all pregnancies occurred in the first three cycles) and very few in the latter cycles (only three pregnancies in the last five cycles).

The first-year pregnancy rate was 4.8 (95%; CI 2.33–7.11) with correct use of the method (pregnancies occurring in cycles in which participants reported no intercourse on Days 8–19). When we include cycles in which women reported intercourse with use of condom or withdrawal during their fertile days, the first-year pregnancy rate is slightly higher (5.7%; CI 3.11–8.16). A 1-year pregnancy rate of 12 (CI 8.47–15.33) was calculated when taking into account all cycles and all pregnancies.

The single-decrement multi-censoring life table for correct use (including only cycles and only pregnancies with no intercourse on Days 8–19) is presented in Table 3. The life table for all cycles is presented in Table 4.

4. Discussion

With only 43 women of 478 in our study becoming pregnant, it appears that the SDM is effective in preventing unplanned pregnancies. As shown in Table 5, efficacy of the SDM is comparable to that of male condoms and is significantly better than that of other barrier methods (female condom, diaphragm, cervical cap, or spermicides) [9].

The finding that the method was used correctly in most cycles (i.e. that couples avoided unprotected intercourse during the entire fertile period as identified by the method)

Table 3
Life table pregnancy rates for correct use of the standard days method

Cycle	Women exposed[a]	Pregnancies	Pregnancy rate	95% confidence interval
1	373	1	0.27	0.00 to 0.79
2	384	2	0.79	0.00 to 1.67
3	361	3	1.61	0.32 to 2.89
4	342	2	2.19	0.68 to 3.68
5	317	0	2.19	0.68 to 3.68
6	297	4	3.51	1.53 to 5.45
7	264	0	3.51	1.53 to 5.45
8	244	2	4.30	2.04 to 6.50
9	242	0	4.30	2.04 to 6.50
10	223	0	4.30	2.04 to 6.50
11	225	0	4.30	2.04 to 6.50
12	215	0	4.30	2.04 to 6.50
13	215	1	4.75	2.33 to 7.11

[a] Excluding censored cycles.

Table 5
Rates of unintended pregnancy during the first year of typical use and the first year of perfect use of user-dependent family planning methods[a] and the standard days method

Method[b]	Pregnancy rate	
	Typical use	Correct use
Chance	85	85
Spermicides	26	6
Cap		
Parous women	40	26
Nulliparous women	20	9
Diaphragm	20	6
Condom		
Male	14	3
Female	21	5
Standard Days Method	**12**	**5**

[a] Source: Hatcher et al. [9].
[b] These figures are drawn from studies using different methodologies, and, therefore, may not be directly comparable.

suggests that those couples admitted into the study were able to understand the method and were capable of translating the method's recommendation into behavior consistent with their expressed reproductive intention. Couples participating in the study seemed no more or no less sexually active than the general population. They reported an average of 5.5 acts of intercourse per cycle. This figure is similar to the 64 yearly (5.3 monthly) acts of intercourse reported for users of coitus-dependent methods in 32 countries throughout the world [10].

Almost all study participants were literate (91% were able to read simple method instructions). No reliable figures are available about schooling in study localities; however, study participants had more years of formal education than their respective national averages.

Participants in the SDM trial are very different from the population of a recent study by Wilcox et al., which reported ovulation as early as cycle Day 8 or as late as cycle

Table 4
Life table pregnancy rates including correct and incorrect use of the standard days method

Cycle	Women exposed[a]	Pregnancies	Pregnancy rate	95% confidence interval
1	452	5	1.11	0.14 to 2.07
2	436	5	2.24	0.86 to 3.60
3	395	8	4.22	2.29 to 6.11
4	363	5	5.54	3.31 to 7.72
5	340	5	6.93	4.41 to 9.38
6	308	6	8.74	5.87 to 11.53
7	280	2	9.39	6.39 to 12.30
8	262	4	10.78	7.52 to 13.92
9	252	0	10.78	7.52 to 13.92
10	236	1	11.16	7.82 to 14.37
11	230	0	11.16	7.82 to 14.37
12	220	1	11.56	8.14 to 14.85
13	218	1	11.96	8.47 to 15.33

[a] Excluding censored cycles.

Day 60. Unlike SDM trial participants, participants in the Wilcox study were neither screened for cycle length before admission to the study nor withdrawn because of cycle length variations (they reported usual cycle lengths from 19 to 60 days) [3]. Many of them clearly would not be eligible to use the SDM.

In designing this study, we were careful to adhere to the criteria for contraceptive efficacy studies defined by Trussell and Kost [7]. Thus, our sample included only women who were likely to be fecund and exposed to the risk of pregnancy. Defining the reason(s) for discontinuation and identifying and reporting early pregnancies detected by laboratory tests also are important. Pregnancies were identified at 42 days post LMP; women who tested negative for pregnancy but who were still amenorrheic were followed until they either menstruated or tested positive for pregnancy.

Most efficacy studies of fertility awareness-based family planning methods do not actually enroll women into the study until they have completed a "learning phase," typically a three-month period during which they receive instruction in the method [11,12]. Pregnancy rates in those studies are artificially reduced if the analysis excludes the early cycles of use. In this study, we included women beginning with their first cycle of use. As previously noted, most pregnancies occurred in earlier cycles.

A weakness of the study was reliance on women's self-reported intercourse and other method use. We expect that women may have under-reported intercourse, especially on Days 8 through 19, and that they may have used other methods (barrier or withdrawal) more frequently than reported. Because the collection of information on intercourse relied on self-reporting, we have no way of confirming the extent of this under-reporting. Another weakness is that the monthly follow-up schedule, while necessary for data collection, may have increased correct use of the method.

Additional questions about the SDM will be addressed in

forthcoming articles, drawing on both additional analysis of the efficacy trial data and from other ongoing research.

5. Conclusion

This efficacy trial demonstrated that the SDM is an effective method of family planning. With a first year pregnancy rate of less than 5% with correct use, it is comparable to other user-controlled methods currently available through reproductive health and other programs. The study also has shown that clients are able to learn the method and to use it successfully to avoid unplanned pregnancy. The SDM offers a valuable addition to the services that reproductive health and other programs can offer. Because it is simple to teach, learn and use, the SDM also has the potential to be provided outside the context of traditional family planning programs, through community development, non-governmental, and social marketing organizations. Operations research studies are ongoing to address some of these issues and explore how best to provide the SDM in these and other settings.

Notes

1. We used Peak day as a proxy for ovulation. Peak day is defined in the Ovulation Method as the last day in a given menstrual cycle on which fertile-type mucus is recognized, or the last day on which the wet or lubricative sensation is felt at the vulva.
2. For ethical reasons, we referred these women for another method because the theoretical protection conferred by Standard Days Method is slightly less for women who consistently have cycles outside the 26 through 32 days range [4]. Although it was explained to them that they were more likely to become pregnant if they continued using the SDM, many of them continued to do so. A further study of these women is ongoing.

Acknowledgments

The authors are particularly grateful to our field collaborators: Dr. Saleg Eid, Catholic Relief Services, Bolivia; Dr. German Coaguila and Pilar Lacerna of Centro de Informacion Educacion y Servicios, Bolivia; Dr. Irma Ramos, CARE, Peru; Beth Yeager, Instituto de Investigacion Nutricional, Peru; and Betty Toledo and Mitos Rivera, Institute for Reproductive Health, Philippines. The Department of Health in Benguet, Philippines, the Ministry of Health in Juliaca, Peru, as well as the providers, researchers, and clients in all study sites made invaluable contributions to this effort. Our special thanks to Drs. James Gribble and James Shelton for their valuable suggestions in the preparation of this article.

The views expressed by the authors do not necessarily reflect the views or policies of USAID or Georgetown University. The Standard Days Method and CycleBeads are trademarks owned by the Georgetown University Institute for Reproductive Health. CycleBeads are U.S. patent pending.

References

[1] Wilcox AJ, Weinberg CR, Baird DD. Timing of sexual intercourse in relation to ovulation. N Engl J Med 1995;333:1517–21.
[2] Wilcox AJ, Weinberg CR, Baird DD. Post-ovulatory aging of the human oocyte and embryo failure. Hum Reprod 1998;13:394–7.
[3] Wilcox AJ, Dunson, D, Baird DD. The timing of the "fertile window" in the menstrual cycle: day specific estimates from a prospective study. Brit Med J 2000;321:1259–62.
[4] Arévalo M, Sinai I, Jennings V. A fixed formula to define the fertile window of the menstrual cycle as the basis of a simple method of Natural Family Planning. Contraception 1999;60:357–60.
[5] Spieler JM, Collins WP. Potential fertility—defining the window of opportunity. J Intl Med Res 2001;29(Suppl. 1):3A–13A.
[6] World Health Organization (WHO). A prospective multicentre trial of the ovulation method of natural family planning. II. The effectiveness phase. Fert Ster 1981;36:591–8.
[7] Trussel J, Kost K. Contraceptive failure in the United States: a critical review of the literature. Stud Fam Plan 1987;18:237–83.
[8] Kazi A, Kennedy KI, Visness CM, Khan T. Effectiveness of the Lactational Amenorrhea Method in Pakistan. Fert and Steril 1995;64:717–23.
[9] Hatcher RA Trussell J, Stewart F, et al. Contraceptive technology. 17th ed. New York: Ardent, 1998;800:Table31–1.
[10] Stover J, Bertrand J, Smith S, et al. Empirically based conversion factors for calculating couple-years of protection. Carolina Population Center 2001:32.
[11] Gray RH, Kambic RT, Lanctot CA, Martin MC, Wesley R, Cremins R. Evaluation of natural family planning programmes in Liberia and Zambia. J Biosoc Sci 1993;25:249–58.
[12] World Health Organization (WHO). A prospective multicentre trial of the ovulation method of natural family planning. I. The teaching phase. Fertil Steril 1981;36:152–8.

Index

A

abortion, 49, 52, 60-61, 64-69, 71-72, 76, 81, 104, 186, 196
abortion, spontaneous, 81
abortifacient, 51
abstinence, 7, 25-26, 30, 36, 38, 43, 66, 108, 142, 150, 152, 170, 174, 182-185, 187, 189-191, 193, 195, 197, 199-213
abuse, 30, 43
acceptability, 111-114, 116-132, 134-136
adolescence, 132, 183-184, 189, 199, 213
adolescent, 7, 12, 69, 132, 184-190, 197-198, 203-207, 209-211, 213
adolescent pregnancy, 184-185, 206
adolescent sexuality, 198, 204
adult, 52, 68, 184, 190, 210-212
adultery, 49
African American, 7, 12, 69, 203-207, 209, 211, 213
African Jamaican, 206
age, 19, 32, 41, 43-44, 64-65, 83, 86, 88-91, 94-98, 102-106, 109, 148-151, 184, 189-196, 205, 210, 219
aging, 6, 8, 11, 101-102, 105
AIDS, 131, 134, 185, 195-196
algorithm, 97, 99, 119, 122, 125, 136, 169, 171-173, 176
amenorrhea, 7, 104, 215, 217-225, 260, 262
American, 4, 7, 12, 69, 76-77, 97-99, 101, 131-133, 135, 165, 176, 203-207, 209, 211, 213, 220-221, 224-225, 246, 265

American Academy of Pediatrics, 221, 224
American Association of Prolife OB/GYNs, 77
American College of Obstetrics and Gynecology, 76, 131
American Society for Reproductive Medicine, 101
anal, 209
anal intercourse, 209
anatomy, 212
androgens, 103, 233
anovulatory, 103, 261
antibody, 235-237
anthropology, 162, 165
antral follicles, 103
Aristotle, 46
artificial birth control, 140-142, 144-145, 149-150, 155, 161-164
artificial contraception, 16, 26, 55, 76
artificial insemination, 76, 84, 98
Asia, 71
assays, 173, 233, 236, 238, 240, 242, 246, 256-257, 260, 265
assessment, 7, 12, 83, 97, 106, 119, 122, 124, 131, 137, 231, 233, 235, 237-239, 241, 243, 245
Augustine, Saint, 43
Australia, 12, 71, 84, 97, 242, 244-245, 264
autonomy, 47, 76, 145, 162
avoid pregnancy, 11, 38, 105, 118, 136, 178

B

babies, 215-216, 218-221, 223-224
barriers, 108, 207, 210

barriers at the fertile time (BAFT), 108
basal body temperature (See BBT)
baptism, 32-33
Barrett and Marshall model, 84, 86, 89
Bayesian model, 85, 87
BBT, 85, 172-173, 175, 242, 254, 256-257
behavioral, 111, 113-114, 141, 164, 183
behavioral change, 113-114
behavioral research, 141, 164
Benedict XIV, 215
Berlin, 228-229
Billings Ovulation Method (See Ovulation Method, Ovulation Method Billings)
birth control, 61, 68, 138, 140-142, 144-145, 149-150, 155, 161-164
Bolivia, 275-277, 280
boyfriend, 151-153, 185
breast, 209, 218, 220, 222-223, 244, 262
breast tenderness, 271
breastfeeding, 7, 12, 215-225
breastfeeding ecological, 7, 12, 215, 217, 219-225

C

calendar rhythm, 137
calendar system, 107
Canadian, 219
Canadian Eskimos, 219
Catechism of the Catholic Church, 15, 18, 20, 27, 71
Catholic, 5, 9-10, 13, 15-18, 20-24, 27, 29, 43-44, 47, 49-50, 55, 57, 67, 71, 74-75, 77, 142, 148, 164-165, 215-217, 227-228
Catholic Church, 15-18, 20, 22-24, 27, 50, 55, 67, 71, 215-216
Catholic Hospital, 74, 77
CCL, (See Couple to Couple League International)
celibacy, 29, 46
cervical, 81, 86, 93-94, 97-98, 172, 175-176, 182, 204, 242, 249, 265
cervical mucus, 81, 86, 93-94, 98, 172, 176, 242, 249, 265
cervix, 83, 172-173, 179-180
charity, 21, 29, 32
chart, 170
charting, 171, 176, 180, 187, 201
chastity, 9, 19, 21-22, 25-27, 30, 36, 52, 75, 183-184, 186, 190, 195-196, 200-202
Chile, 222
childbearing, 133, 150
childbirth, 41, 52, 217-219, 221, 265
children, 20, 23, 29-30, 32, 39, 41, 49-50, 56, 59-60, 63-66, 68-69, 103, 120-121, 123, 186, 208, 211, 219
child spacing, 217-220, 224
choice, 7, 57, 64-65, 73, 105, 113, 116, 149, 195, 209, 212, 227-229
Christ, 10, 18, 31-34, 39, 42-43, 48
Christian, 19, 27, 29-30, 32-33, 35, 39-40, 44-46, 148, 206, 211
Christianity, 39
Christi fideles laici, 31, 33
Church, 9-10, 15-24, 26-27, 29-31, 33, 41, 43, 49-50, 55-56, 67-68,

Index

71, 77, 148, 206, 212, 215-216, 227
church attendance, 148, 206
civil law, 72
Civil Rights Act, 53
Clearplan Easy Fertility Monitor™ (118, 125, 131, 135, 137, 263
Clomid, 104
Clomiphene Challenge Test (CCT), 104-105
cloning, 49, 65
cohabitation, 16
commitment, 74, 114, 209, 212-213, 228
communion, 20, 22, 31, 37-38
communication, 11, 25-26, 33, 41, 43, 69, 116-117, 122-126, 130, 132-137, 139-145, 147, 150, 152-154, 156-161, 166-168, 179, 243, 248
community, 12, 19, 25, 32-33, 64, 136, 166, 168, 184, 186, 200, 207
conception, 6, 66, 79-95, 97-99, 119, 125, 131, 138, 165, 169-171, 174, 176-177, 182, 208, 218-219, 225, 262
conceptual analysis, 111, 122
condom, 60, 117, 123-124, 131, 136
condom use, 117, 131
confidence, 55, 87, 122, 135, 142, 175
conscience, 5, 10, 54-55, 66, 71-72, 74, 76-77, 227
continuum, 241, 243, 245, 257, 260-264
control, 23, 43, 54, 57-61, 64, 67-68, 102, 120-121, 132, 135, 138, 140-145, 149-150, 153-155, 158-159, 161-164, 166, 170, 183-184, 188-190, 192, 195, 198-199, 201, 264
contraception, 5, 7, 10, 12, 16, 22, 26, 30, 38, 49-61, 63, 65-67, 71, 74, 76-77, 102, 107, 110-112, 114, 116, 131-133, 137-139, 164, 166-168, 170, 186, 196-197, 227, 229-230, 263
contraceptive, 43, 50-52, 54-56, 58-60, 77, 83, 97, 116-118, 121, 132, 141, 145, 149-150, 152-153, 155-159, 162, 167-168, 184, 186, 190-191, 228
contraceptive coverage, 50-51
contraceptive devices, 51, 60, 97
contraceptive drugs, 50-52, 55, 58, 60
contraceptive efficacy, 118, 121
correct method use, 275, 279-280
corpus luteum, 103, 248, 253-254
Council of Affiliated Menopause Societies, 272
couple, 7, 10, 12, 21, 25, 30-42, 47, 57, 59, 65, 82, 86-87, 105, 115-116, 118-120, 122-127, 130, 132-138, 141-142, 144-145, 147, 154, 159, 161, 164, 167-168, 180, 182, 215, 219, 224
couple communication, 116, 124, 126, 130, 134, 141, 144, 147, 154, 159, 161, 167-168
Couple to Couple League International (CCL), 180, 217
covenant, 18, 34-35, 37-38, 40, 44
Cracow, 228-229
creation, 17, 23-24, 32, 38-39, 59, 111, 123, 138, 186
Creator, 26-27, 33, 36, 42-43

Creighton Model, 84-85, 93, 95, 98, 109
Creighton Model Fertility Care™ System, 84
culture, 15-16, 32, 39, 43, 46, 49-50, 55-56, 76, 78
Cue, 170-172, 176-177, 179
cycle, 6, 8, 10, 12, 22, 24-25, 58, 60, 64, 79, 81-83, 85-89, 91, 93-99, 103-105, 119, 122-126, 128-130, 145, 163, 170-175, 178, 181, 188, 190, 196, 218, 228, 231-235, 237-239, 243, 246-251, 253-257, 259-264
CycleBead™(s), 107, 276-277, 280
cycles, irregular, 102, 104

D

day specific probability of conception, 79, 81-92, 94
decision, 53-54, 65-66, 114, 116, 198, 227
decision-making, 25, 134-135, 212
demographic, 24, 79, 97, 144, 154, 159, 161, 166, 228
Depo-Provera, 77
diocese, 6-7, 166, 200
diocesan, 5, 9, 11-13, 75, 142, 164, 166
Diocesan Development Program (DDP), 9, 13, 75, 142, 164
divorce, 49, 148
disease, 38-39, 54, 63, 65, 67, 74-75, 131, 195, 198, 204, 224
doctor, 51, 62-63, 65-66, 73, 217, 219
Dunson model, 85, 87-89, 93

E

Ecclesia in America, 33, 44

education, 7, 18-19, 22-23, 61, 72-73, 75, 131, 147-149, 153, 155, 157-158, 160, 183, 185-187, 189, 191, 193, 195, 197-202, 216, 228
effectiveness, 11, 25, 72-73, 79, 97, 107-109, 114, 171-172, 174, 181, 186
efficacy, 6, 8, 74, 107-108, 110, 118, 121-122, 125, 176, 183, 186, 204
egg, 80
electrolyte, 169-171, 175-176, 178
embryos, 65, 80
end of marriage, 21
endometrium, 225
endocrinology, 98, 246, 264-265
England, 84-85, 88, 98, 118, 177, 182
environment, 68, 79, 94, 257
enzyme, 235, 237, 246, 265
epidemiology, 225
Equity in Prescription Insurance and Contraceptive Coverage (EPPC) (bill), 51
Erickson v Bartell Drug Company, 53, 61
estimated day of ovulation, 81, 85, 88-89
estradiol, 103-104, 248-251, 253
estrogen, 83, 85, 93, 103, 188, 239, 242, 253-254, 261
estrogenic Mucus, 82
estrone glucuronide (E1G) 232-245, 249, 253, 255-263
ethical, 16, 71, 73-75, 80, 227, 229
ethics, 7, 27, 44, 71, 77, 227-228
Ethical and Religious Directives, 71, 74
Ethiopia, 117, 133
Eucharist, 31-33, 39

Europe, 71, 76, 85, 118
European, 84, 88-91, 93, 95, 118, 121, 125
Evangelium vitae (See Gospel of Life)

F

faith, 1, 3, 5-6, 8-9, 13, 15-19, 21, 23-27, 33-34, 41, 49, 211-212, 215
faithful, 22, 30-31, 55, 74, 77, 208
fallopian tubes, 80
Familiaris Consortio, 20, 22, 27, 38
family, 1, 3, 5-13, 15-27, 29-32, 40, 43-44, 47, 49-50, 54, 56, 60, 62, 65-67, 72-74, 77, 79, 97, 99, 102, 105, 107-112, 118, 120-121, 124, 131-132, 134-144, 147, 149-152, 154, 156, 160-161, 163-165, 167, 169-170, 176-177, 182, 197-198, 200, 205-207, 210-211, 215-216, 219, 224-225, 227-229, 231, 244, 246-247, 249
family planning, 1, 3, 5-9, 11-13, 15-18, 20, 22-27, 29-30, 49-50, 54, 56, 60, 65, 67, 72-74, 79, 97, 99, 102, 105, 107-110, 112, 118, 121, 124, 131-132, 134-144, 147, 149-152, 156, 160-161, 163-165, 169-170, 176-177, 182, 197-198, 215-216, 224-225, 227-229, 231, 246-247, 249
Family Practice, 77, 139-140, 144, 147, 167
family size, 25, 60, 121
Family of the Americas Foundation (FAF), 6, 139, 147-149, 151-153, 155, 158, 160-161, 163
father, 31-32, 187, 200-201, 211
fatherhood, 29

FDA, 51, 170, 178
fecundability, 82, 84, 86-87, 90-91, 93-95, 97-98, 102, 105
fecundity, 11, 21, 89, 95, 98, 105
feeling like an object, 139, 141, 154-156, 158-161, 163, 166-168
Federal Employee Health Benefits Program, 51
female, 10, 12, 35, 37, 39, 42, 50, 53, 58, 60, 62-64, 66, 81-82, 89, 97-98, 105, 114-115, 122, 130, 135, 188-190, 197, 204-205, 247, 249
fertile, 26, 38, 58, 64, 81-83, 86-94, 108, 169, 172-176, 178-182, 232, 234-235, 239-240, 243-247, 253-254, 256-257, 260-265
fertile phase, 178-182, 232, 240, 257
fertile window, 81-83, 86-90, 93-94, 169, 172-176, 180-181, 234, 239, 247, 256
fertility, 7-8, 10-12, 20, 23-25, 35-36, 38-39, 41-42, 50-51, 54, 56-60, 63-64, 66-67, 74-76, 79, 84, 86-90, 93-99, 101, 103, 105-106, 114-116, 118, 120-121, 125-127, 129, 131-132, 135-138, 141-142, 144-145, 161-163, 165, 169, 171-179, 181-184, 186-188, 190, 192, 198, 200-202, 217-221, 227-228, 231, 235, 241-243, 245-249, 253-256, 258, 260, 262-265
fertility awareness, 10, 58, 60, 75, 142, 187-188, 192, 198, 200-202
fertility appreciation, 58, 60, 137, 188
fertility monitor, 7, 12, 84, 118, 125-126, 131, 135-137, 169,

171, 173, 175, 177-178, 242, 246, 263, 265
fertility regulating methods, 114, 116
fertilization, 65, 76, 80, 97-99, 105-106
fetal, 52, 65, 76, 102
fetal experimentation, 52
fetus, 64-65, 72
fidelity, 19, 21, 33-34, 37-38
follicular, 95, 102, 175, 232-233, 235, 242-243, 248, 256, 265
follicular phase, 232-233, 235, 242, 256
follicle, 93, 102-103, 233, 235, 248-251, 253, 255, 260-263
Follicule Stimulating Hormone (See FSH)
folliculogenesis, 93
Food and Drug Administration, 52
framework, 10, 32, 37, 113-114, 132, 140, 164
freedom, 21-22, 35, 37, 74, 76-77, 241
freedom of conscience, 74, 76-77
frequency of intercourse, 89, 150, 155, 157-158, 160
FSH, 103-106, 248-249, 251, 260

G

Gaudium et spes, 15, 17, 19, 21, 27
gender, 189, 204
Genesis, 23, 40
genetic, 65, 80-81, 90
genetic factors, 80-81
genital, 38, 186-187, 209, 247, 249
Georgetown University Institute for Reproductive Health, 11, 107
Germany, 7, 12, 84, 95, 118, 227

gift, 10, 20, 23, 26, 31, 35, 37-39, 58-59, 137, 202
girl, 26, 187-188
girlfriend, 210, 212
God, 17-20, 23, 26-27, 31-32, 34, 36, 38-39, 42-44, 47, 58-60, 67, 69, 136, 143, 202, 212, 215-217, 220, 223
gonadotropin, 80
Gospel, 32-33, 39, 216
Gospel of Life (Evangelium vitae), 218
granulosa cells, 103, 250, 253
Gregory the Great, 215
Gynecologist, 11

H

health, 6, 9-11, 21, 24-27, 40-41, 50-58, 61, 65-67, 72-74, 76, 79, 93, 96, 99, 102, 107, 111, 131, 172, 176, 185, 198, 206, 213, 225, 231, 233, 238, 254, 257
health benefit, 50-51, 53
health care, 9, 24, 51-52, 54-55, 61, 66, 72-74, 76
heath care delivery, 72-73
health insurance, 50-51
high-tech method, 108
Hispanic, 131, 148
HIV, 132, 184, 196, 201, 204
holistic, 9, 20-21, 136
holistic health, 9, 21
Holy Spirit, 34, 42
hope, 10, 12-13, 17, 29, 32-33, 76-77, 138, 181, 201, 221, 231, 241
hormone, 80, 95, 110, 131, 169, 172, 178, 201, 235, 239, 242, 244, 248-249, 253-254, 259-260, 262-263

Index

hospital, 10, 26, 40, 69, 74, 77-78, 96, 137, 185, 208
hot flashes, 103-104
human, 8-9, 12, 16-27, 30, 34-35, 37-40, 42-44, 46-47, 49-52, 55-60, 67-68, 71-72, 79-80, 94-98, 102, 140-141, 144, 161-162, 164-165, 167, 177, 183, 200, 202, 205, 208, 212, 216, 224, 227-228, 231, 246-247, 264-265
human chorionic gonadotropin (hCG), 80-81, 88
human cloning, 49
human dignity, 49, 55
human fertility, 51, 58-59, 79, 97, 202
human life, 16, 38, 49, 55-56, 59, 68, 71
human person, 9, 18, 20-24, 26, 39, 43-44, 141, 161-162, 164
human reproduction, 58, 94-96, 177
human sexuality, 18, 20-24, 27, 42, 47, 49-50, 55-56, 58-59, 67, 183, 200
Humanae vitae, 22-23, 27, 57-59, 61, 165, 216-218
husband, 22, 26, 60, 115-117, 134, 151-153, 167, 216, 219
hypothalamic-pituitary-ovarian axis, 241, 269

I

illness, 40-41, 67
immunoassay, 246, 265
implantation, 80
income, 148-149, 153-155, 157-160, 167, 186, 206
infallibility, 16
infant, 215-216, 222, 224-225
infertility, 54, 56-57, 63-64, 79, 84, 90, 93, 98, 102, 104-105, 118, 134, 137-138, 170-171, 181, 215, 217, 219-220, 222-224, 240, 242, 245, 262
Inhibin A, 103
Inhibin B, 103
insomnia, 103
insurance, 50-52
instrument, 170-172
integrity, 19, 21, 24, 76, 78, 145, 161, 164, 228
intercourse, 11, 18, 23, 30, 33-34, 36-39, 41, 64, 66-67, 80-89, 91, 93, 97-98, 126-127, 144, 150, 152-153, 155, 157-160, 173, 177, 182, 184-186, 189-190, 198, 203, 206, 209, 241-242, 244-245, 256
interpersonal communication, 145, 160
intimacy, 20, 26, 36, 42, 134-136, 139-140, 142-143, 164-165, 209
Intra Uterine Device (See IUD)
in vitro fertilization, 65, 76, 99
irregular cycles, 102, 104
IUD, 52, 109, 135

J

Japan, 137
Jesus, 29, 31-32, 39-40
John XXIII, Pope, 59
John Paul II, Pope, 22, 31, 37-39, 140, 165

K

kingdom, 26, 32, 95, 118
kingship, 31, 39-41, 46

284   Index

knowledge, 17, 75, 84, 122-124, 128-130, 134-136, 138, 187-188, 190, 201, 203, 219, 231, 243

L

lactation, 7, 12, 215, 218-219, 222, 224-225, 265

Lactation Amenorrhea Method (LAM), 7, 12, 215, 217-219, 221-223, 225

laity, 29, 31, 47

La Leche League, 218

language of the body, 37, 39, 41-42

law, 9, 19, 23, 27, 44, 50, 52, 55, 65, 72, 216

legal, 10, 50, 52, 63-64

legislation, 51-52

LH, 102-103, 118, 169, 172-173, 175, 178-179, 240, 248-249, 252-253, 257, 261

libido, 103

life, 7, 10, 13, 16-22, 25, 27, 29-33, 36, 38-44, 46-47, 49-50, 55-59, 68, 71-72, 76, 81, 102, 120, 135-136, 138, 143, 148-150, 162, 186-187, 200, 203, 205-207, 209-211, 213, 216, 220, 222, 225

limiters, 134, 244

litigation, 53

love, 19-22, 26, 33, 35-38, 40-45, 47, 50, 58, 69, 113, 140, 142, 144, 165, 188, 209, 211, 224, 227

London, 95, 131-132, 238-239, 254

Lumen gentium, 29, 31, 47

luteal, 234, 239, 243, 245, 254, 256, 262

luteal phase, 234, 239, 243, 245, 254, 256, 262

luteinizing hormone (See LH)

M

Magisterium, 30, 215

male, 37, 39, 42, 58, 62-63, 81-82, 114-115, 122, 129, 132, 134, 185, 188-190, 197, 201, 204

man, 18, 20-21, 23, 33, 38, 40, 43, 59, 63, 67-69, 90-91, 114

manipulation, 37, 41, 58, 72, 163

marital, 5-6, 10-11, 19, 25-27, 29-31, 33-35, 37-39, 41-43, 45-47, 135-137, 139-145, 147, 149, 151, 153-155, 157-161, 163-167, 216, 227-228

marital act, 216, 227

marital chastity, 25-27

marital satisfaction, 6, 11, 139-145, 147, 149, 151, 153-155, 157-161, 163-167

marital sexuality, 42-43

marriage, 16-21, 24-26, 29-35, 37, 39, 42-44, 46-47, 49, 52, 151-152, 165, 187, 192, 200, 202, 204, 211

MaterCare International, 71

maternal, 76, 89, 211, 215-216

Maternal Fetal Medicine, 76

maturity, 19, 21, 184, 186, 190, 210

maximum probability of pregnancy, 94

medical ethics, 71, 77

medical profession, 25, 56-58, 65

medical residency (See residency)

medical schools, 71

medical students, 71, 77

medicine, 10, 51, 57, 60, 62, 65-66, 71, 74, 76, 78-79, 97, 101, 182, 227

Melbourne, 97, 238, 244-245, 256, 263-264

menarche, 102, 246, 262, 264
menopause, 63, 102-105, 263
menopausal transition, 104, 114
menses, 64, 102, 104-105, 119, 239
menstrual, 6, 8, 12, 79, 81-83, 85-89, 91, 93-99, 103, 118-119, 122, 171, 178, 188, 231, 245-249, 251, 254, 257, 264
menstrual cycle, 6, 8, 12, 79, 81-83, 85-89, 91, 93-99, 103, 231, 246-248, 251, 257, 264
menstruation, 80, 188, 217-218, 222-223, 225
metabolites, 83, 249, 251
method, 6-8, 11-12, 24-26, 35-36, 41-42, 84-85, 97, 99, 105, 107-112, 114, 117, 120-124, 127, 132, 134-137, 141-142, 149, 156, 158, 161, 165, 169, 171-180, 182, 215, 217-218, 222, 224-225, 244, 246, 249, 255, 257, 264
method efficacy, 108
method effectiveness, 25
method pregnancy rate, 108
Mexican, 117
midwife, 76
mind, 17, 20, 24, 57, 67, 163, 182
miscarriage, 81, 104
monitor, 7, 12, 65, 67, 84, 118, 120-129, 131, 135-137, 169, 171, 173, 175-178, 187, 231-246, 249, 253-258, 260, 263-265
morality, 7, 16, 22, 55, 76, 227-229
mother, 26, 40, 62, 186-187, 200-201, 210, 215-221, 223, 225
motherhood, 29, 63
Mother Theresa of Calcutta, 40
mucus, 81-83, 85-86, 88, 93-95, 98, 103-104, 172-174, 176, 179-180, 182, 187, 233-235, 239-242, 244, 249, 254-257, 261-262, 265
mucus symptom, 94, 180, 233-235, 239-242, 254-256
Mulieris dignitatem, 42
mutual respect, 25
mutuality, 41, 145

N

nadir, 170
National Institute on Aging, 269, 272
National Institute of Child Health and Human Development, 269, 272
National Institute of Environmental Health Sciences, 6, 79, 172
Natural Family Planning (See NFP)
natural law, 216
nature, 17-18, 30, 34, 38, 41, 47, 51, 57, 60, 64-65, 67, 114, 116, 118, 123, 162, 216-217, 220-221, 227, 236, 260
New Testament, 41
New Zealand, 7-8, 12, 84, 231, 247, 264
NFP, 5-6, 9-13, 17, 19, 21, 23, 25-27, 30-31, 33-39, 41-43, 45, 47-48, 51, 53, 55, 57-61, 66-67, 71, 73, 75, 77, 79-82, 84, 94, 105, 108-109, 134-145, 147, 149-161, 163-176, 178-182, 200, 215, 229-231, 241-245, 247, 249, 257, 260-261, 263
NFP only-physician/OB/GYN, 78
night sweats, 103
non-virgin, 183, 189, 192-196
North American Menopause Society, 269

North Carolina (data set), 84-85, 88, 93
nurse(s) (as in professional nurse), 72, 75-76, 222
nursing (as in breastfeeding), 9, 12-13, 62, 72, 215, 218-224

O

OB, 76-77
object, 54, 72, 139-141, 145, 147, 150-151, 153-161, 163-164, 166-168
object, feeling like an, 139, 141, 154-156, 158-161, 163, 166-168
obstetrics, 5, 10, 65, 69, 71, 73, 75-76, 78, 98, 105, 131, 225, 227, 246, 264-265
obstetrician, 11, 217
obstetrician gynecologist, 11
oral contraceptives, 63, 135, 138
- (See also contraceptive, birth control, artificial contraception)
oocyte, 102
ova, 90, 98, 254
OvaCue™, 169-176, 178-182
ovary, 8, 102, 239, 247-249, 251, 253, 255, 257-259, 261, 263, 265
ovulation, 24, 81-89, 93-94, 96-99, 103-104, 125, 169-173, 176-182, 187, 218, 224, 234-235, 239, 243-247, 250, 252-253, 255-257, 259, 261-265
ovulation method, 24, 84, 97, 99, 176, 179-180, 244, 255
Ovulation Method Billings, 84, 244, 255
Ovarian Monitor, 7, 12, 84, 231-237, 239-241, 243, 245-246, 249, 253-255, 257-258, 263-265
ovulatory cycle, 234-235, 254-257, 261-262
ovulatory phase, 81, 102, 175, 263

P

pacifiers, 219-221
parent, 37, 68, 187, 206
parenthood, 25, 32, 42, 66, 69
patient, 63, 65-67, 69, 73-74, 76, 104, 132
Paul VI, Pope, 57, 95
Peak Day of Mucus (also Peak Mucus Day), 81, 85, 180, 233-235, 240-242, 254, 256-257, 261
peer, 185, 199, 201-203, 212
peer pressure, 203, 212
perimenopause, 6, 101-102
perinatology, 76
periodic continence, 10, 22, 30-31, 35-36, 41
person, 9, 15, 18-24, 26, 32, 35-37, 39-40, 42-44, 46, 52, 58-59, 65, 137, 140-141, 145, 161-164, 195, 201, 208-210, 216, 227, 245
Persona(, 108, 118-126, 135-136, 200
personhood, 142, 144, 162-163
Peru, 271-274, 275-277, 280
Philippines, 271-274, 276
philosophers, 36, 68
physical, 20, 24, 31, 36, 41, 47, 55, 58, 60, 138, 186, 209, 213, 217
physician(s), 66-67, 71-75, 77, 98, 170
physiological parameters, 6, 101
physiology, 80, 82, 209, 213, 247
pill(s), 52, 56, 66 (See also artificial contraception)
Pius XII, Pope, 225
Planned Parenthood, 66, 69

Political, 18, 49
Pope Paul VI Institute for the Study of Human Reproduction, 95
population, 16, 23-24, 82, 86, 92, 97-98, 105, 118, 131-132, 138, 166, 168, 183-184, 190, 208, 241
Populorum progressio, 23, 27
Postmenopause, 271-272
prayer, 34, 36, 69, 212
practice, 5-7, 10, 12, 22, 25, 30-31, 39, 41-43, 47, 59, 69, 71-77, 80, 104, 139-144, 147, 149-150, 152, 160-161, 163-165, 167, 170, 172, 175, 203, 216, 221, 231, 233, 235, 237, 239, 241, 243, 245
pregnancy, 6, 11, 30, 38, 41, 47, 49, 52-54, 63-64, 72-73, 79-83, 85-90, 94-98, 102-105, 108-109, 111, 113, 115, 117-119, 121, 123, 125-127, 129, 131-134, 136-137, 144, 150, 174, 177-178, 181-186, 190, 195-198, 200, 202, 206, 213, 217, 222-223, 244, 246-247, 254, 257, 262-265
pregnancy rate, 108
Pregnancy Discrimination Act, 53-54
Pregnanediol glucuronide (PdG), 233-241, 243-245, 249, 253-254, 256-263
premarital, 150, 184, 189-190
premarital pregnancy, 184, 190
premarital sex, 189
prescriptions, 51, 55
priest, 10, 31, 46-47, 67
priesthood, 33-35, 46
primacy, 145
primordial follicles, 102
probability, 81-83, 86-91, 93-94, 98, 177, 182

probability of conception, 81-82, 86-88, 90-91, 93, 98, 177, 182
procreate, 20, 186
procreation, 18, 22-23, 186
progesterone, 83, 85, 104, 187-188, 248-249, 253-254
proliferative phase, 102
prophecy, 31, 37, 46, 129
prophet, 10, 31, 40, 46
Protestants, 228
post-ovulatory, 171-172, 240, 256, 260, 263
puberty, 63, 207
public policy, 49-50, 52, 54, 197

Q

quality, 36, 86, 88, 95, 116-117, 119, 122, 124, 172, 176, 249

R

radioimmunoassay (RIA), 237-240, 246, 264
relationship, 15-17, 20, 30-32, 36, 40-42, 74, 79-80, 91, 97, 115, 117-120, 122-124, 126, 128, 135-137, 141-145, 150-153, 155, 159, 162-168, 187, 189, 210-211, 224-225, 265
religion, 7, 16, 53, 148-149, 206, 227-228
religiosity, 143-144, 155, 158, 160, 211
religious, 9, 16, 46, 54, 59, 71, 74, 148-149, 153-154, 157, 160, 166-167, 185, 195, 206, 209, 211, 227-229
religious attendance, 148-149, 153, 157, 160, 166
Religious commitment, 228
religious hospitals, 74

reproduction, 58, 94-96, 105, 177, 209, 257
reproductive, 6, 8, 11-12, 66, 77, 79-82, 101-104, 107, 109, 122-124, 126-127, 130-131, 134-136, 170, 212, 257
reproductive aging, 6, 8, 11, 101
reproductive anatomy, 212
reproductive capacity, 79-80, 82
reproductive health, 11, 107
reproductive knowledge, 122-124, 134-136
reproductive physiology, 80, 82
research, 6-7, 10-12, 17, 25, 49, 52, 55, 68, 79-80, 82-83, 88, 95, 97, 107, 111-112, 131, 135, 139, 141, 143-145, 147, 159-160, 164, 167-168, 172, 197, 200-202, 205, 208, 213, 217-219, 231, 233, 235, 237, 239, 241, 243, 245-246, 260, 265
residency, 65, 74, 77
residency training, 74
responsibility, 18, 20, 22-23, 25, 45, 117, 126, 135, 142, 165, 196-197, 209, 246, 264
rhythm, 22, 137
right to life, 72
risk factors, 200

S

sacrament, 18-20, 33, 43-44
salivary, 170, 176, 178
Sanger, Margaret, 69
Schwartz model, 85-88
science, 1, 3, 5-6, 8-9, 13, 15-19, 21, 23-25, 27, 72, 94, 101, 105, 107, 131, 215, 224-225, 246, 264-265

Second Vatican Council, 15, 17, 29, 31
self, 117, 188, 207, 210
self-centered, 212
self-control, 134, 142, 144
self-esteem, 117, 139-140, 142, 164-165
self-giving, 21, 33, 36-37, 44, 145
self-knowledge, 183, 188, 190, 196
self-mastery, 21, 135
self-worth, 122, 135
sex, 30-32, 35-36, 38-39, 41, 43, 46-50, 53, 55-56, 58-59, 66, 98, 116, 120, 132-133, 150, 154, 177, 182-186, 189-190, 192, 195-198, 200-202, 204, 208-211
sex - before marriage, 49, 192
sexual, 10, 18, 23, 26, 30-31, 33-43, 46, 48, 56, 66-67, 69, 81-82, 97-98, 116-117, 127, 131-136, 144, 150, 152-162, 177, 180-188, 190-192, 195, 197-198, 200-206, 208-209, 211-213
sexual abstinence, 43, 152, 187, 203-205, 208-209
sexual abuse, 30, 43
sexual activity, 46, 66, 127, 153, 180-181, 183, 190-191, 197-198, 200-204, 211-212
sexual intercourse, 18, 23, 33-34, 37, 39, 66-67, 81, 98, 144, 152-153, 159, 177, 182, 184-186, 198, 203, 206
sexual intimacy, 134, 136
sexual pleasure, 117, 132, 135-136, 161
sexuality, 7, 18, 20-24, 27, 41-47, 49-50, 55-56, 58-59, 67, 142-143, 183, 185, 187, 189, 191, 193,

Index 289

195, 197-202, 204, 207, 209-210, 212-213
Sexually Transmitted Infections, 63, 203
Sexually Transmitted Diseases (STD), 184, 196
shared responsibility, 135, 142
signs, 24, 75, 80, 144, 171-172, 175, 178, 181-183, 247
sin, 34, 211, 215
Smith, Janet, 49
society, 10, 16, 18-19, 23-24, 27, 56, 59-60, 64-66, 101, 141, 202, 221, 224, 228
sociology, 11, 139
soul, 20, 24, 26-27, 67, 77, 164, 216
spacers, 134, 244
sperm, 80-82, 86, 88, 90, 93, 99, 242, 247
spirit, 23, 31, 33-34, 42
spiritual, 5, 9, 19-21, 24, 29-31, 36-37, 42-43, 47, 136, 142, 164-165, 203, 209
spiritual well-being, 136, 142, 164-165
spirituality, 5, 29-31, 33, 35, 37-39, 41-47
spousal, 139-141, 144-145, 147, 150, 152, 154, 156-161, 167
spousal communication, 139-141, 147, 150, 152, 156-161 (see also communication)
spousal support, 147, 150, 152, 154, 156-161, 167
spousal supportiveness, 139, 141, 150, 159-160
spouse, 36, 41, 47, 139, 145, 147, 150, 153, 155-159, 161, 163

Stages of Reproductive Aging, 6, 8, 11, 101
Standard Days Method (SDM), 107-110, 271-276
statistical, 79, 83, 85-86, 89, 93, 99, 108, 122, 143-144, 147, 158, 167, 175, 219
statistical models, 85
STD (See sexually transmitted diseases)
sterilization, 71, 76-77, 102, 109, 135, 137-138
stem cell, 49, 52
sub-fertile, 83, 93-94
supportive, 142, 145, 152, 160
survey, 131, 138, 142-143, 147-148, 151-153, 163-164, 167, 185, 191, 198, 219, 224
Sympto-thermal Method, 84-85, 109, 169, 173, 175, 179
symptoms, 93, 97, 102-104, 173, 185, 234, 243-244, 247, 257, 263

T

technology, 11, 16, 65, 75, 108, 126, 132, 134, 137, 178
teen, 11, 183, 186-189, 191, 197-202, 204, 206, 211
Teen Star Program, 11, 183, 186, 200, 202
teen pregnancy, 186, 197-198, 200, 202
teenage pregnancy, 205
teenager, 66, 185-186, 214 (See also adolescent, teen)
theology, 9-10, 44, 46, 48, 165
theology of the body, 44, 165
theologians, 29-30, 227
time to pregnancy, 82

timing of intercourse, 80, 98
Title VII, 53
thecal cells, 103
theory, 42-43, 141, 166-168, 184, 190, 235, 263
totality, 22, 24, 26, 36, 38, 145, 162, 227
transmission of life, 21-22, 57
trust, 25, 119, 121, 144-145, 182
Two Day Method (TDM), 109
Type E estrogenic (mucus), 82
typical-use pregnancy rates, 108

U

ultrasound, 95, 250-251, 265
United Kingdom, 95, 118
United Nations International Children's Emergency Fund (See UNICEF)
United States, 5, 9-10, 13, 25, 27, 44, 71, 75-76, 84, 118, 121, 125, 142, 198, 213, 221
United States Conference of Catholic Bishops (USCCB), 5, 9, 13, 27, 71, 75, 164
UNICEF, 221, 223, 225
unintended pregnancy, 132, 174
unwanted, 63, 111, 123, 183, 195-196
unwanted pregnancy, 63, 111, 123, 183, 195-196
urinary hormones, 108
US Chamber of Commerce, 50, 52, 61
US Senate, 52, 61
uterine lining, 80
uterus, 65

V

vagina, 209

vaginal dryness, 103
vaginal intercourse, 209
values, 10, 17, 19, 21, 26, 36, 42, 111, 140-141, 144-145, 151-153, 156, 159, 161-164, 187, 197, 209, 235, 238-240, 243-245, 254-258, 260-263
Vatican (II) (See Second Vatican Council)
virgin, 46, 183, 189-190, 192-196
virginity, 183-184, 190, 198
viability, 81, 90, 98-99
vocation, 20, 32-33, 38, 40-41, 46
Von Hildebrand, Dietrich, 36, 45
vulnerability, 40, 74

W

weaning, 221, 245
well-being, 16, 19, 23, 36, 136, 139-140, 142, 144, 164-165
wife, 22, 26, 38, 115-116, 216
withdrawal, 37, 104, 108, 261
women, 6, 10-12, 29, 32-33, 39, 49-51, 53, 55, 58, 60, 62-68, 72, 74, 80-81, 83-85, 89-90, 93, 96-98, 101-105, 109, 111, 117-121, 123, 125-126, 128-129, 132, 135, 138-139, 141, 143-145, 147-153, 155-157, 159, 161-172, 175, 178-179, 186-188, 204-205, 209, 211, 214, 219, 228, 233, 237-238, 241, 244, 254, 256-257, 263
women's health, 65, 96, 111
World Health Organization (WHO), 25, 93, 99, 131, 233
World Federation of Catholic Medical Associations (FIAMC), 71
worth, 84, 110, 213, 260

Y
youth, 46, 185, 187, 191, 198-204, 209, 212-213